PENGUIN BOOKS

THE COT DEATH
COVER-UP?

Jim Sprott is a highly respected consulting chemist
and forensic scientist. During his wide-ranging
career he has been involved in forensic work
relating to some of New Zealand's most famous
criminal cases. In 1995 he was awarded the OBE
for services to forensic science and the community.
He has been researching the cause of cot death for
over fifteen years.

THE
COT
DEATH

COVER-UP?

Jim Sprott

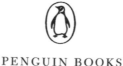

PENGUIN BOOKS

PENGUIN BOOKS

Penguin Books (NZ) Ltd, 182–190 Wairau Road, Auckland 10, New Zealand
Penguin Books Ltd, 27 Wrights Lane, London W8 5TZ, England
Penguin USA, 375 Hudson Street, New York, NY 10014, United States
Penguin Books Australia Ltd, 487 Maroondah Highway, Ringwood, Australia 3134
Penguin Books Canada Ltd, 10 Alcorn Avenue, Toronto, Ontario, Canada M4V 3B2

Penguin Books Ltd, Registered Offices: Harmondsworth, Middlesex, England

First published by Penguin Books (NZ) Ltd, 1996

1 3 5 7 9 10 8 6 4 2

Copyright © T J Sprott, 1996

Designed and typeset by Egan-Reid Ltd, Auckland
Printed in New Zealand

Contents

List of Graphs

Foreword

This is a book for parents everywhere, but particularly parents in the western world, where cot death is a scourge. It provides the answer to the conundrum of cot death. Not a medical answer, because cot death isn't a medical problem. It is a problem of environmental chemistry.

It is fondly believed in some quarters that New Zealand leads the world in cot death research. It doesn't. The answer to cot death has come out of Britain.

New Zealand's prime contribution to cot death research has been some excellent epidemiology – but epidemiology only describes cot death. It doesn't explain the cause. This book does.

The focus in New Zealand on epidemiology rather than the cause of cot death is the reason why the New Zealand cot death rate is no longer falling. The New Zealand Cot Death Association have known since 1991 about the research which is the basis of this book, but they simply ignore it.

I expect this book to be roundly criticised by the orthodox cot death establishment. It isn't written in highly technical language, it isn't clogged up with references to learned journals, and – probably worst in their eyes – it isn't 'peer-reviewed'.

But this book isn't aimed at academics. It is aimed at parents – parents who can't understand why avoiding risk factors doesn't stop cot death; parents who pray every night that their baby will still be alive in the morning and who lie awake listening for its breathing; and parents for whom, sadly, it is already too late.

It is written in the hope that parents, doctors, midwives, childcare workers – maybe even academics – will read it, and that as a result the lives of babies will be saved.

T J Sprott OBE
MSc PhD FNZIC
Auckland
NEW ZEALAND

June 1996

Introduction

C ot death (Sudden Infant Death Syndrome, or SIDS) is the biggest environmental disaster this century. It occurs almost exclusively in Western Europe, North America and Australia. Although we do not know precisely how many babies have died of cot death since it was first defined in 1953, the figure is about one million. The number of deaths caused by disasters like Bhopal and Minamata pales in comparison.

Because it is spread over a huge population in many countries and over such a long time, cot death doesn't seem like an environmental disaster. It doesn't grab the headlines or cause public outrage or political fallout. It just continues, year after year, one death at a time, a seemingly random occurrence. Nevertheless, cot death is a direct result of environmental pollution.

In 1986 I arrived at the conclusion that cot death was due to inadvertent and unsuspected gaseous poisoning by an extremely toxic nerve gas generated by microbiological action on something within the baby's cot; but I could not identify the gas.

In 1989 Barry Richardson, working independently in Britain, came to the same conclusion and in addition identified the gases. His finding confirmed my original hypothesis.

The poisonous gas arises from the mattress where the baby sleeps. It is formed by the action of a common and otherwise harmless household fungus on certain chemicals within the mattress itself. This finding, which is now known as the Richardson hypothesis, explains every known factor concerning cot death, and also provides a simple means of eradicating it.

Since its first publication in Britain, not a single valid criticism of the hypothesis has been put forward.

By contrast, research in New Zealand into the cause of cot death is in the doldrums, and it has been in the doldrums for years. Some useful epidemiology has confirmed factors which increase the risk – including placing babies in their cots face down, overwrapping them, prematurity, and low birth weight. A greater incidence of cot death has been noted among lower socio-economic groups.

Warnings about risk factors, especially prone sleeping, have reduced cot death in New Zealand, but the rate remains distressingly high, especially among Maori. Despite the partial success, no progress has been made in New Zealand by established cot death researchers in determining the actual cause of cot death or the mechanism whereby the risk factors increase its likelihood.

The Richardson hypothesis was first made public in Britain in mid-1989 and the cot death rate there started to fall immediately.

Nevertheless the New Zealand Cot Death Association will not admit even the possibility that the hypothesis may be correct.

At the political level, letter after letter to the New Zealand Ministry of Health draws only perfunctory acknowledgement or a restatement of the position held by the New Zealand Cot Death Association. Overseas the pattern is similar.

And all the while, appeals such as Red Nose Day come around each year.

There are some bright notes. A number of orthodox cot death researchers appear to be softening their views towards the hypothesis. Several talkback radio stations have co-operated in putting it before the public. After all, surely parents have the right to know about this research so they can make their own decisions.

But there will be no real progress in eliminating cot death in New Zealand, or elsewhere for that matter, while present official policies and attitudes remain.

For too long cot death has been regarded as a medical problem. But the cause doesn't lie in medicine. It lies in environmental chemistry, microbiology and toxicology.

This research is not just theoretical: since the hypothesis was first publicised late in 1989, the British cot death rate has plummeted. It is now about one quarter of the rate in New Zealand.

New Zealand's cot death rate continues to be the worst in the world.

Acknowledgements

W hen a book relates to an issue of broad public interest, the thanks to be recorded range far and wide. For their technical input and dogged persistence in the search for the cause of cot death, and for the extensive data which they placed at my disposal, my sincere thanks go to Barry Richardson and Peter Mitchell, both of Winchester, England. I am indebted to Peter Muller OBE, of Invercargill, New Zealand, for his valued assistance with my early research in Southland; and to Joan Shenton, Ron Rooney and the *Cook Report* team in Britain for the information which they provided. I wish to record my special thanks to The Baby Factory in New Zealand for their generous donation of cot bedding for analysis; and to the many cot death mothers, healthcare professionals, parents and grandparents in both Britain and New Zealand who have offered encouragement and shared their experiences. Finally, I express my appreciation to friends and colleagues who have shown interest in this project; to my daughter, Alison, who transposed my chemist's style into readable English; and to my wife, Marion, for her support throughout.

1

Inspiration in Britain

S ummer 1988. In the leafy suburban precinct of Lainston Close near the ancient cathedral city of Winchester, a family wedding was being celebrated. The bride was the daughter of unassuming British consulting scientist Barry Richardson and his wife Janet. On the lawn was a large marquee where speeches were made, toasts were drunk and merriment prevailed.

The Richardsons had hired the marquee from Mitchell Marquees. Peter Mitchell, proprietor of the marquee company, is an ebullient entrepreneur living in Winchester, where he has various business interests. In his early days – doing a reverse Grand Tour – he visited New Zealand and for a while worked on the construction of the Auckland Harbour Bridge. Now in his sixties, he specialises in the manufacture and hiring out of marquees and other outdoor amenities. He's good at it. So good, in fact, that he has even supplied equipment for the Wimbledon Tennis Tournament and the Farnborough Air Display.

It has always seemed to me that Peter Mitchell was an unlikely person to stumble upon the cause of cot death, but that is what he did. And it all came about unexpectedly.

Soon after the wedding Barry and Peter, both members of the Rotary Club in Winchester, were sitting together at lunch. When Peter learned that Barry was a consulting scientist specialising in preventing the degradation of materials, he was immediately interested. He had a problem with his marquees and awnings. They were made of heavy PVC (polyvinyl chloride) plastic, and deterioration was occurring: after a short period a fungal growth appeared, causing unsightly staining. Peter asked Barry to investigate the problem and tell him how to overcome it.

Barry's reply was that no investigation was needed: the staining was caused by a common fungus which became established in the plastic, consuming the plasticiser in the PVC as a food source.

(PVC is a rigid plastic, hard and brittle, and not widely used in this form. The familiar flexible sheeting is rendered pliable by the introduction of plasticisers, of which there are several types. The most common types used in ordinary PVC sheeting are called 'external plasticisers'. These are low volatility organic solvents which are mutually soluble in the PVC. As more of the plasticiser is blended with the original PVC, the sheeting becomes more tough and flexible.)

Peter took Barry's answer back to his PVC supplier, who told him the problem could be overcome by increasing the amount of biocide in the PVC, thus killing the fungus. A biocide is a material which prevents the growth of micro-organisms. Biocides used in PVC are frequently based upon the toxic element arsenic and are added to plastics intended for use in the tropics. The actual compound which the PVC supplier was using was OBPA (oxybisphenoxyarsine).

The supplier's suggestion was vetoed by Barry, who explained: 'The biocide won't kill this fungus – instead, the fungus will consume the biocide as well as the plasticiser. Since the biocide contains arsenic, the fungus will generate a very poisonous gas which would be harmful to your staff working with the marquees.'

The PVC supplier listened politely to Barry's warning but didn't accept it.

Not knowing who to believe – Barry or his PVC supplier – Peter contacted the OBPA manufacturer in Austria, whose reply was even stronger: Barry was talking nonsense and OBPA was perfectly safe. And then came the crucial remark: 'It's even approved for use in babies' mattresses.'

Peter pondered on this reply and at about midnight that night woke suddenly with the thought: if Barry is right and the supplier is wrong, could this be the cause of cot death? As soon as it was dawn, he phoned Barry. 'Yes, it could be,' said Barry, 'and I'll even name the fungus for you: it's probably *Scopulariopsis brevicaulis.*'

On this note started the research programme which finally elucidated the answer to cot death, a problem which had confounded medical researchers worldwide, consumed millions of research dollars, and caused the deaths of so many infant children. The research destroyed the conventional wisdom that cot death has many causes, gave the answer to every known factor about cot death which epidemiologists had discovered, and also provided a cheap and immediate means of eliminating it.

2

The Concept of Poisoning is Born

My interest in the cause of cot death was kindled in the early 1980s. There had been much publicity on the topic – how the rate in New Zealand was the worst in the world – and how the rate in Southland was by far the worst in New Zealand, about double that in the North Island.

The strong seasonal variation had been reported, the rate rising with the approach of winter, peaking in August and September and then falling off rapidly. There had not been any publicity about the benefits of face-up sleeping – that would not appear for several years – but a number of possible causes of cot death and lines of research were advanced, all based on medical grounds.

I had no personal contact with cot death, nor did I know anybody who had, but my interest as a scientist was aroused. It just didn't make sense. Here we were, living in a prosperous country with a well-educated population, enjoying advanced medical care and all the benefits of organisations such as Plunket. Yet we also had the worst cot death rate in the world. Not only this, but the worst was in Southland.

It didn't add up. Southland is a prosperous region, stable, conservative, inhabited in large part by careful people of Scottish descent – the sort of people who don't take risks. But in Southland by the mid-1980s the cot death rate was approaching 10 deaths per 1000 live births, and during the winter could rise to double this rate. In one neighbourhood in Invercargill, in just one residential block, five babies died of cot death during one winter. It had reached the stage where babysitters and grandparents minding children didn't watch the TV – they watched the baby, and were relieved when the parents arrived home.

The Southland cot death rate was far higher than that in Britain, for example, or British Columbia or Scandinavia. Yet these were very similar societies to Southland in terms of race, climate and standard of living. It was quite apparent that these disparities in cot death rates could not be explained on medical grounds.

Another fact seemed inexplicable on any medical hypothesis. Cot death on this scale was a new phenomenon. It had suddenly surged in the 1950s and was rising steadily. If you talked to older parents and grandparents about cot death, they typically replied, 'We never heard about it in our day.' Babies then died of diphtheria, or whooping cough, or other illnesses – but they didn't just die.

The sudden increase in babies' deaths was so inexplicable that it was even suggested that parents had now begun to deliberately suffocate their babies. The population just didn't know what to make of it.

By the mid-1980s it was clear that, despite all their research, medical investigators had no idea of the cause of cot death. There had been some suggestion overseas that babies lying face down in their cots were more at risk of dying, but this proposition was hotly denied by other researchers.

As a scientist, I was convinced that there must be some logical explanation, if only I could think of it. My thought pattern went like this:

Cot death babies clearly were not ill and didn't die of any illness. If there had been a pattern of illness causing cot death, the medical researchers would certainly have found it – but they hadn't. Equally, it was inconceivable that this rise in unexplained deaths was due to suffocation, either accidental or deliberate. Accidental suffocation was known to be extremely rare, and I was not prepared to believe that so many parents had suddenly started murdering their babies. There was only one possible conclusion: since the babies were not ill, and since they were not being suffocated, they were obviously being exposed to some poison. There was no other rational explanation.

I first published this idea in 1986. By then I had become convinced that cot death was due to unsuspected and inadvertent gaseous poisoning, and that the poison arose from something within the baby's cot.

That changed the whole complexion of the matter. It took the cause of cot death out of the field of medicine or any 'mechanical' factors and put it squarely in the field of environmental chemistry and toxicology. The shift of emphasis from medical thinking to that of chemistry brought cot death into the scope of the most logical and predictable of sciences. I realised then that if this line of thought were followed, the cause of cot death would eventually yield to logical thought. The solution would be found as a result of a full understanding of the chemistry of the baby's environment.

At this point I couldn't envisage what the poisonous gas might be, so I started looking at chemicals to which babies were exposed; and discovered – as it would turn out – a contributing factor to cot death (but not the cause).

Babycare in New Zealand by the mid-1980s had become almost an art form. New products saturated the market, babycare magazines were appearing, and new mothers were bombarded with promotions and free product samples even before they left the maternity ward to bring their baby home. All the 'old-fashioned' methods of babycare went out the window. Instead of soap, the new mother was told to use 'modern' detergents; instead of boiling nappies, bottles and teats, she was told to sterilise them in chemicals. She was told that good mothering required the baby's surroundings to be made sterile, and that only chemical sterilants could achieve this end. Just washing clothes and bedding wasn't good enough for baby – she must ensure 'extra bounce and softness' with fabric softeners.

And like many new mothers, she listened to the modern propaganda, keen to be up-to-date. She loaded up her baby's environment with a cocktail of substances totally foreign to the environment of babies born before the 1950s. And the cot death rate soared.

By contrast, in British Columbia where I was living at the time, baby laundry was washed in a pure soap powder and there were no nappy soaks or bottle and teat soaks on the market. And interestingly, while cot deaths occurred there, I noted that the rate was about three times lower than in New Zealand. Was there a connection, I wondered. And would the New Zealand cot death rate fall if mothers went back to 'old-fashioned' methods?

Here Southland came back into the picture. It had all the advantages and requirements for a particular study. As an isolated community of largely European descent, it was not subject to sudden shifts or influences from other regions. The stable population would be ideal for carrying out trials and collecting data. Their level of education and conservative approach meant that research forms would be filled out carefully and consistently.

In addition to these features, there was another incentive for focusing these ideas on Southland: the *Southland Times* newspaper, highly regarded throughout the region, widely read, and under the competent editorial control of forward-thinking Peter Muller.

The plan was to publicise and promote radical changes in babycare and then monitor the results. If there was anything in the environmental poisoning idea, it should show up quickly in Southland.

Peter Muller and I had been friends for some time. I had often sent him letters and other newspaper copy, which he frequently published, so I approached him with the idea of a babycare questionnaire and trial. He took it up enthusiastically. The programme was introduced as a front page news item, which in itself guaranteed almost saturation publicity. Parents were invited to phone in for a questionnaire form and the *Times* sent them out at its own expense. The completed questionnaires were couriered to me in Canada and I set about analysing the data.

Sixty Southland families who had lost a baby to cot death responded to the questionnaire, representing most of the cot deaths which had occurred in Southland over the previous few years; 218 families who had not lost a baby to cot death also completed the questionnaire.

The results confirmed my suspicion: the use of all the modern chemical synthetic babycare products was very widespread in Southland. Of those families who had experienced a cot death, 76% were using synthetic detergents, 83% were using chemical nappy soaks and 74% were using chemical soaks for bottles and teats.

This came as no surprise. It is well known by international marketing companies that New Zealand is a soft touch for the promotion and evaluation of new products. Nationwide advertising is easy and cheap to carry out and products are quickly taken up by an appreciable number of people. The marketing successes and failures show up rapidly and products can be readily abandoned or adjusted accordingly for sale in bigger countries. In marketing parlance, New Zealand is regarded as a test market area and it seemed that this sort of promotion had happened with babycare products. (Interestingly, such products had not reached the North American market.)

Young mothers, of course, are a vulnerable group where marketing is concerned, desperately keen to do everything right for their babies. In a community such as Southland, with relatively good incomes and education, and lacking the statistical dilution of Polynesian babycare practice, it was predictable that use of the heavily promoted synthetic chemical products was almost endemic.

Among non-cot death families, however, the results were quite different. Only 34% of these families were using synthetic detergents for baby laundry. Only 45% used chemical nappy soaks, and of those who did, almost all then put them through a full washing machine cycle. Furthermore, as few as 23% of non-cot death families were sterilising bottles and teats with chemical soaks.

It was December 1988 and time to visit Southland. If the

use of these products could be discontinued during early 1989 in time for the usual winter upsurge in cot death, any impact on the cot death rate brought about by changes in babycare would become apparent by December 1989.

Again, Peter Muller gave me total support, and so did the local television and radio stations. Mothers were advised to stop using detergents and synthetic soaking solutions, and to wash babies' clothes and bedding with soap and without fabric softeners. They were told not to soak bottles or teats in chemicals, but instead to boil them. The local branch of the Cot Death Association was furious with me, but I went back to Canada and waited.

From various snippets which reached me, it was clear that many mothers took note of what I had recommended. Peter sent me the Southland cot death statistics from time to time during 1989 and I could scarcely believe what was happening. By the end of the year Southland had gone from having the highest cot death rate in New Zealand to the second lowest (bettered only in New Plymouth). From 23 cot deaths in 1987, and 13 in 1988, only 5 were recorded in Southland in 1989.

Not only that, but in the neighbouring Canterbury and Otago regions, where my recommendations had received some publicity, the rate had also fallen. (In Otago not one cot death occurred in the five months following the announcement of my recommendations in December 1988.) By contrast, the rate in Auckland, where the recommendations were not published, increased markedly.

During this same year the cot death rate in the rest of New Zealand had risen, but Southland's rate had come down from an average of 8.5 per 1000 live births over the three years 1986–1988 to 2.8 per 1000 in 1989.

This result was far beyond my expectations and warranted attention by the authorities. During a visit to New Zealand in the latter half of 1989 I put the provisional results of the Southland trial before Helen Clark, then Minister of Health, and Don

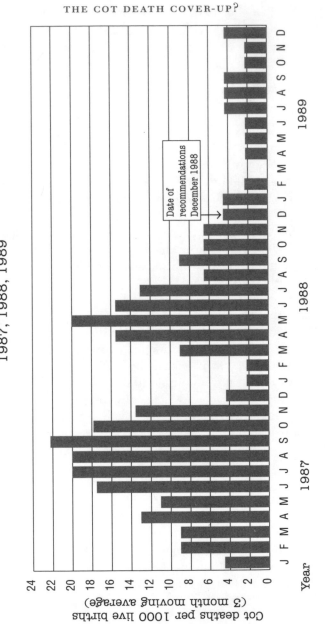

COT DEATH RATES IN SOUTHLAND, NEW ZEALAND
1987, 1988, 1989

Cot deaths per 1000 live births
(3 month moving average)

Date of
recommendations
December 1988

Year   1987   1988   1989

Data: Southland Area Health Board

22

COT DEATH RATES IN SOUTHLAND, NEW ZEALAND 1987, 1988, 1989

This graph shows the remarkable results which were achieved during 1989 in Southland following the 'back to basics' campaign. Parents were advised to wash babywear in soap rather than detergent and not to use fabric softeners or nappy sterilants; baby feeder bottles and teats were to be washed clean and then sterilised in boiling water; any milk stains on bottles and teats were to be rubbed off using dry salt.

For the three years 1986–87–88 the cot death rate in Southland had averaged 8.5 per 1000 live births, probably the highest rate ever recorded anywhere in the world.

The 'back to basics' recommendations were widely publicised throughout Southland during December 1988. The rate during 1989 fell from the highest in New Zealand to the lowest except for New Plymouth. The actual reduction was from 8.5/1000 to 2.8/1000. During 1989 the rate in the North Island increased to about 4.5/1000.

The Southland publicity had also spread to the neighbouring regions of Otago and Canterbury and a sharp reduction in the 1989 cot death rate was noted in these regions as well.

McKinnon, then Opposition health spokesman.

There was no doubt in my mind that the clue to cot death lay somewhere in the chemistry of the baby's environment, but just what it was, I did not know.

3

There's Nothing New . . .

I did not claim as a result of the Southland study to have discovered the cause of cot death, but it was apparent that something of significance had happened. As I would realise later, I had detected what is now referred to as a 'risk factor': a set of circumstances which renders a baby more likely to succumb to the prime cause of cot death.

The 'cot death establishment' of medical researchers shrugged off the results, but they couldn't explain the success of the Southland trial or the simultaneous reduction in the number of cot deaths in Otago and Canterbury. Nor could they be encouraged by the 1989 cot death statistics for the rest of the country. They chose to ignore the Southland study.

According to Dunedin Medical School researcher, Dr Barry Taylor, the Southland figures were 'natural variation', meaningless unless consistent for at least three years and accompanied by a reduction in the use of chemicals. In fact, the Southland rate *did* stay down (though during 1990 the benefits of face-up sleeping had also received some publicity), and Dr Taylor informed me that sales of the babycare products in question had slumped.

Dr Shirley Tonkin (now national co-ordinator of the New Zealand Cot Death Association) made a remark about 'people without a scientific background' getting involved in cot death research. But she still told a newspaper reporter that, in her opinion, the products were a waste of money and that they probably didn't do babies any good.

Felicity Price, regional co-ordinator for the Canterbury Cot Death Society, said she was delighted with the reduced

Canterbury figures but couldn't explain why the change had occurred. Her delight didn't stop her from making three complaints to the New Zealand Press Council regarding publicity given to my research.

(Some years later, the New Zealand Cot Death Study group would publish a paper saying that the use of nappy sterilants wasn't a 'risk factor'. They based this claim solely on epidemiology but in my view there was a flaw in their logic. As shown by the graph on page 136, some of their results demonstrated that the use of sterilants seemed to be a risk factor.)

In the context of New Zealand in the 1980s – a time when modern products were automatically assumed to be better than those they had replaced, and when marketing claims made by big companies were largely accepted – it was radical to suggest that mothers should go back to basics and that chemicals readily available on the market might be dangerous. But actually there was nothing new in this sort of discovery.

In the nineteenth century in Europe there was an explosion in the knowledge of chemistry, and with it a host of new products to enhance the everyday life of an increasingly affluent society. Examples are legion, but prominent amongst these products were new dyestuffs and pigments. Brilliant new colours such as the aniline dyes were suddenly available for women's clothes, curtains, wallpapers and carpets, for decorating houses, and for colouring paint. Nowadays we take these things for granted, but when they appeared on the market they revolutionised fashions and home decoration.

One beautiful colour was extremely popular for home decoration in the latter half of the nineteenth century. It came in two forms, Scheele's green (named after the outstanding German chemist) and Paris green, the French equivalent. However, it was derived from copper arsenate, and that caused a problem.

During that period thousands of children died unexpectedly throughout Italy, Germany, France and Britain. Many adults also were made ill, but no-one could explain what was happening. These were days of prevalent illness and high child mortality, but this was something else again. The medical profession of the time was totally mystified and suspicions of foul play arose.

There had been unexplained reports of poisoning from volatile compounds of arsenic since the 1820s and the typical 'garlic-like' odour of these gases had been noted. In 1874 the Italian chemist F. Selmi first associated this odour with the presence of mould and suggested that a mould was generating the gas arsine from arsenical compounds. But not until 1892 was the source of the poison discovered: it turned out to be the new arsenical pigments which had been so enthusiastically adopted. Another Italian chemist, B. Gosio, noticed the unusual garlic odour in rooms where children had died and adults had become ill, and he recognised this as the odour which he had regularly encountered when testing for arsenic. 'Gosio's arsenic' was the name given to the extremely toxic gas which was coming from wallpaper and carpet coloured with Scheele's green.

Gosio proved that the arsenic in these pigments was converted into gas by a fungus known at the time as *Penicillium brevicaule*. Then it was discovered that 'white arsenic' (arsenious oxide), added as a rodent repellent to wallpaper adhesive produced from horse hooves, was also a source of poisoning.

It was a brilliant and significant finding at the time and led to the establishment of the 1901–1904 British Royal Commission on Arsenical Poisoning. A century later its significance would be rediscovered.

Instances of the poisoning which led to Gosio's finding recurred from time to time over subsequent years. In 1932 some British children in the Forest of Dean, playing under a house where concrete blocks contained arsenic, died from Gosio's arsenic (although by this time the gas had been identified as arsine and closely related gases).

Perhaps the best known instance this century was in 1947, when Mrs Clare Booth Luce, United States ambassador to Italy, nearly died from arsenical poisoning. She too was exposed to Gosio's arsenic, arising from green pigment in the paint on her bedroom ceiling in the embassy in Rome.

Technology moved on, and Gosio's arsenic and, more important, its mode of formation, was forgotten – except among a few chemists. One such chemist was Barry Richardson, whose knowledge of this early example of the mechanism of chemical poisoning led him to solve the cot death conundrum.

Perhaps even Gosio and some earlier nineteenth century chemists were not the first to know about the hazard of gas arising from the walls of houses where there was some arsenic. A very intriguing passage appears in the Bible in Leviticus, Chapter 14, where the Israelite people were given certain instructions regarding their houses if mildew (in some versions referred to as a spreading leprosy or a plague) was found on the inside walls. The text refers to a fungal growth described as greenish or reddish (the latter being the colour of *P. brevicaule*, now known as *Scopulariopsis brevicaulis*). If mildew was found, the priest was instructed to scrape it off and examine the house again after seven days. If the growth had ceased, the people could return to the house, but if not, the house had to be broken up and taken out of the city to be disposed of.

This passage in Leviticus may refer to different hazards arising from micro-organisms, but it is known that the mortar used in those days by all the tribes of the region and later by the Romans was what we call 'pozzolana', a natural cement. Pozzolana was derived from volcanic regions, where soils frequently contain arsenic. The growth of the mildew could therefore have generated arsine (or trimethyl arsine) with deadly results, especially for children.

The common moulds are of the *Aspergillus* variety, *niger* (black) and less frequently *flavus* (yellow). It is noteworthy that there is no warning in Leviticus against moulds of these colours. Such moulds are harmless and do not give rise to toxic gases.

4

Some Basic Chemistry

There are 92 elements naturally occurring on earth, some in very large amount and others barely detectable. Noble metals like gold and silver have been known from antiquity. Iron was an early discovery, as were lead, tin and other base metals. To the early chemists, the elements they discovered one after another seemed to have neither rhyme nor reason.

The science which we know today as chemistry began with the alchemists, who for centuries kept up a fruitless endeavour to convert base metals into gold. Their work was not without value, because they discovered the properties of many elements and compounds. But how the seeming mishmash of elements and information fitted together remained a mystery until a Russian scientist, D. I. Mendeleyev, discovered in the late 1860s that there was a logical progression from one element to the next, and that elements could be categorised in groups according to their similar properties.

From this momentous concept (which other chemists had also been formulating for some time) was developed the Periodic Table of the Elements, which is reproduced in part on page 31.

The elements which are important to this narrative all fall into Group Vb of the Periodic Table. The first two members of the group, nitrogen and phosphorus, are well known; but the remaining three, arsenic, antimony and bismuth, are rarely encountered in normal daily life.

Arsenic and antimony were known to the ancient world. They are usually described as 'metalloids', meaning that they look like metals but are hard and brittle and their chemistry falls between that of the typical true metals (such as lead and copper) and the non-metals (such as carbon and sulphur).

Antimony was known to the Romans as *stibium*, and this name persists in many languages to this day.

Bismuth, a brittle greyish-white metal, was discovered in 1780.

Nitrogen is a gas, comprising about 80% of the earth's atmosphere. To early chemists the concept of a gas was difficult, and it was not until 1772 that nitrogen was identified as an element.

Phosphorus, another relatively recent discovery (1674), is a waxy solid, although it is seldom seen in this form. It has one peculiarity: it glows in the dark, which accounts for the derivation of its name from the Greek words *phos* (meaning light) and *phoros* (bringing).

These elements may appear to have no connection, but in fact they do. They all belong to Group Vb because they have similar electron structures. (It is on this basis that the elements in the Periodic Table are assigned to their respective groups.)

The chemistry of any element depends on its electron structure, and consequently all the Group Vb elements form similar compounds. In particular, they all form hydrides (compounds between the element and hydrogen) of the same type. The first of these hydrides, the hydride of nitrogen, is the well-known gas, ammonia. The hydrides of the remaining elements in Group Vb are little known: they are phosphine, arsine, stibine (from antimony) and bismuth hydride.

Phosphine, arsine and stibine all share a significant characteristic: they are among the most poisonous gases known, about a hundred times more poisonous than hydrogen cyanide and a thousand times more so than carbon monoxide. Their toxicity is comparable with that of Sarin (related to phosphine), the modern nerve gas which was used in the Iran–Iraq war in the 1980s and the Tokyo subway episode in 1994. The degree of toxicity of these gases is almost beyond mental comprehension.

SECTION OF THE PERIODIC TABLE
OF THE ELEMENTS

V/Vb

+3 5 **B** 10.81 2-3	+2 ±4 6 **C** 12.011 2-4	±1 ±2 ±3 +4 +5 7 **N** 14.0067 2-5	−2 8 **O** 15.9994 2-6	−1 9 **F** 18.998403 2-7
+3 13 **Al** 26.98154 2-8-3	+2 ±4 14 **Si** 28.0855 2-8-4	±3 +5 15 **P** 30.97376 2-8-5	+4 +6 −2 16 **S** 32.06 2-8-6	±1 +5 +7 17 **Cl** 35.453 2-8-7
+3 31 **Ga** 69.72 -8-18-3	+2 +4 32 **Ge** 72.59 -8-18-4	±3 +5 33 **As** 74.9216 -8-18-5	+4 +6 −2 34 **Se** 78.96 -8-18-6	±1 +5 35 **Br** 79.904 -8-18-7
+3 49 **In** 114.82 -18-18-3	+2 +4 50 **Sn** 118.69 -18-18-4	±3 +5 51 **Sb** 121.75 18-18-5	+4 +6 −2 52 **Te** 127.60 -18-18-6	±1 +5 +7 53 **I** 126.9045 -18-18-7
−1 +3 81 **Tl** 204.383 -32-18-3	+2 +4 82 **Pb** 207.2 -32-18-4	+3 +5 83 **Bi** 208.9804 -32-18-5	+2 +4 84 **Po** (209) -32-18-6	±1 +5 +7 85 **At** (210) -32-18-7

N = nitrogen
P = phosphorus
As = arsenic
Sb = antimony (stibium)
Bi = bismuth

And it was these gases which unexpectedly turned up in Barry Richardson's cot death research.

The toxicology of a gas comprises two concepts: the lethal dose and the mechanism by which the gas is poisonous. Phosphine, arsine and stibine vary somewhat as regards their toxicity, arsine being the most poisonous, followed by phosphine and then stibine.

The lethal dose of such poisonous gases is usually expressed as that quantity which will kill half of the exposed population within a certain time. It is very difficult to assess the lethal dose of phosphine, arsine and stibine in relation to babies. First, the gases are extremely uncommon, never arising normally in the household environment. Secondly, they are more dense than air and tend to settle to the floor, where they are less readily detected. Thirdly, they are relatively unstable and will quickly decompose in the air after they are generated.

Nonetheless figures have been published for the maximum allowable limits of concentration of the three gases for adults. For occupational exposure the USA threshold limit value (TLV) for phosphine is 0.4mg/cubic metre of air (0.3 parts per million); for arsine 0.15mg/cubic metre (0.05ppm); and for stibine 0.5mg/cubic metre (0.1ppm). These limits vary slightly from country to country. For example, in Sweden the limit for stibine is 0.3mg/cubic metre (0.05ppm).

The approximate lethal dose of stibine for babies over a 30 minute exposure has been calculated at 1 milligram per cubic metre of air. To put this amount into everyday perspective, this weight of gas equates with the amount which a household aerosol would deliver into the air in a burst lasting one-thousandth of a second. Thus it will be seen that a minute amount of stibine is sufficient to render one cubic metre of air lethal to a baby.

A baby breathes approximately 35 times per minute and each breath takes in about 20 millilitres of air. Therefore a baby breathes in about 700ml per minute. One cubic metre contains 1000 litres (= 1,000,000ml), which is the amount of air a baby would inhale over a period of nearly 24 hours. Since, however, it is known that a cot death can occur within 1 hour, the actual amount of stibine involved can be as little as 0.02mg. (The amount for phosphine is even less.)

The mechanism of poisoning for phosphine, arsine and stibine is the same. They are described as being 'anti-cholinesterase agents' and, like many other gases with this property, are termed 'nerve gases'.

To understand the term 'anticholinesterase' it is necessary to discuss how nervous impulses pass from the brain to various organs such as the heart and lungs. Nerve pathways are a series of short disconnected nerves joined together by synapses, and an impulse leaving the brain must be transferred from one short nerve to the next. This transfer is effected by the conversion of a molecule of the substance choline (always present in the body) to acetylcholine. The acetylcholine in one nerve end stimulates the next nerve in order to transmit the impulse. But for successive impulses to travel along the nerve, the acetylcholine must first be destroyed, and for this purpose our bodies contain an enzyme called cholinesterase.

If the blood is poisoned by a substance which de-activates cholinesterase (an anticholinesterase agent), the vital process of destruction of acetylcholine does not occur. The result is a build-up of acetylcholine in the blood. This affects the central nervous system by inhibiting the passage of brain impulses from travelling along the nerve to the organ concerned. If, for example, the organ in question is the heart, the outcome will be erratic heartbeat and finally cessation of heart function. Likewise, if impulses are prevented in this way from reaching the lungs, breathing becomes irregular and then stops.

It is well known that phosphine, arsine and stibine are anticholinesterase agents. There is, however, an important difference between the speed at which such anticholinesterase agents affect, respectively, adults and infant children. In the case of an adult, the first effect is a headache, resulting from depression of the central nervous system, and after some hours' exposure partial destruction of the blood, leading eventually to death. Of course, adults react to a headache and take some action to alleviate it. If they are sleeping, they will wake up long before any serious harm is done.

Infants, on the other hand, are less able to help themselves. Older babies, if they get a headache while in their cots, will throw off blankets, stand up and generally draw their parents' attention to their distress. However, babies under six months old are too small to do these things. They may become fractious, but they appear to be very sensitive to the gases and succumb quickly.

Heart and respiration functions are controlled by the vagus nerve, but infants are much more dependent than adults on the autonomic nervous system, which acts to maintain a steady state within the body's internal environment. In infants the anticholinesterase process rapidly causes cardiac inhibition and thus cot death can ensue.

In 'near miss' cases, the heart stops but is restarted. Nevertheless the intervening failure of the blood supply to the brain can result in brain damage, sometimes serious.

The increased sensitivity of infants to anticholinesterase agents is borne out by the fact that, unlike adults who die from phosphine, arsine or stibine poisoning, cot death babies do not exhibit haemolysis (the decomposition of substances in the blood). The lack of haemolysis in cot death babies has been advanced as an argument that cot death is not caused by these toxic gases. But this argument overlooks the fact that anticholinesterase activity causes babies to die *before* haemolysis (a relatively slow process) can occur and therefore this convenient diagnostic feature is not present. The greater sensitivity of children to accidental phosphine poisoning is reported in the literature.

Furthermore, the mechanism of cot death as a result of cessation of nerve function to the heart and lungs is borne out by the records of monitors, devices used by parents to maintain a check on their baby's breathing and heartbeat. These event monitors often show a progressive decrease in heart rate before breathing stops, which is exactly the sequence one would expect from poisoning by an anticholinesterase agent.

There are now many reports of cases where cot death has been attributed to heart failure brought about by abnormality of the vagus control of the heart muscle but post-mortem examination has not revealed any such abnormality. Significantly, these symptoms describe precisely the result of failure of the vagus system due to poisoning by the anticholinesterase action of phosphine, arsine or stibine.

As to the source of the gases in a baby's environment, antimony, which used to be common in British cot mattresses, is sometimes present in New Zealand mattresses and frequently present in sheepskins. Antimony has certainly resulted in many cot deaths in Britain and there is a strong indication that it has done so in Western Europe and North America.

Stibine, which derives from antimony, has a garlic-like odour but it is a very dense gas, over four times heavier than air. Thus an adult tending a baby in its cot would not normally notice the characteristic odour of stibine because the gas would be flowing off the mattress and falling to the floor.

In New Zealand phosphorus is more common than antimony in mattress materials. It seems invariably to be present in sheepskins, and can also occur in fabric coverings and synthetic foam fillings, as well as in ti-tree bark and various natural and synthetic padding materials.

Phosphine, which derives from phosphorus, is an insidious gas. It is essentially odourless and extremely toxic. In one known case in Britain a family of two adults and two children was killed by phosphine at a concentration of about 1.5ppm. Phosphine leaves no trace in the body, although there is sometimes congestion in the lungs. It is not much heavier than air, and in the warmth around a sleeping baby its density could easily reduce to about that of the surrounding air. Thus it will remain in the environment of the baby and at the low concentrations involved will not be detectable by smell.

Arsenic is present in some sheepfleece wool. It arises naturally where sheep are grazed on volcanic and mineralised soils (a common circumstance in New Zealand and certain parts of Australia) and is excreted into the wool. It is also used commercially as a biocide to protect certain plastics against mould attack in the tropics. At one time British Army-issue cot mattresses contained an arsenical biocide, but this practice was discontinued when the danger to babies was publicised.

Arsine, which derives from arsenic, is the best known of the three gases and appears to be the most toxic. It too has a garlic-like odour, which tends to protect adults against poisoning, but the lethal dose for babies seems to be extremely low. It is considerably heavier than air, so that the odour would not normally be noticed by an adult tending a baby.

In terms of quantities of the three elements likely to be encountered in cots, the amounts present are frequently far greater than would be required to produce a lethal dose of the respective gases. For example, in Britain even in the 1990s concentrations of antimony and phosphorus in the range of 1% or more have frequently been found in cot mattress components. To put this in perspective, 100 grams of such mattress material would contain 1000mg of one or both of the elements. As calculated above, the lethal dose, when converted to the gas, is for a baby about 0.02mg. This means that the area of mattress beneath a baby, say 300 grams, would contain 15,000 times the amount of the element required to produce a lethal dose.

The gas could not all be liberated at once, of course, and it is conceded that these calculations are only approximate, but the point is clear: if any of these elements are naturally present in or have been added to cot mattress material, the amounts are likely to be considerably more than those needed to produce dangerous levels of phosphine, arsine or stibine.

5

A Strange Fungus – Benign and Deadly

We are surrounded by a myriad of micro-organisms. They are in the home, in the garden, in much of the food we eat and in our bodies. People loosely call them microbes or germs, words which have acquired – quite wrongly – the connotation of 'harmful'. In fact, some micro-organisms are essential to life.

Some *are* harmful, such as *Salmonella typhimurium*, which brings on food poisoning; *Staphylococcus aureus*, which causes infections in wounds; *Mycobacterium tuberculosis*, which infects the lungs; and many more. Yet the harmful organisms make up only about 3% of all known species.

Many micro-organisms are useful. A number of them decompose dead plants and animals, recycling vital elements back into the soil. They are also used in the treatment of sewage, converting pollutants into products such as nitrates and phosphates. The micro-organisms which normally inhabit our bodies – called our microflora – protect us from many disease-causing micro-organisms.

We also use micro-organisms in the manufacture of foods such as cheese, yoghurt, beer, wine and bread. Micro-organisms such as *Bacillus thuringiensis* are used to combat insects which would otherwise attack food crops.

Broadly speaking, micro-organisms are divided into several groups: viruses, bacteria, fungi, protozoa and algae. Fungi are further divided into yeasts and moulds.

Moulds are very common and are often seen in the household environment, for example, on foodstuffs, and on fabrics which have been stored in a damp condition. Sometimes they are found on wood and concrete under houses where there is dampness.

Most moulds are multicellular. The cells join together to form long thin filaments called hyphae. As these hyphae grow, they branch and intertwine, producing a visible colony, or mycelium. Some of the hyphae rise above the substrate on which the mould is growing, forming structures called spores, from which the moulds propagate.

A particular feature of mould spores is that they can survive very harsh circumstances such as heat, cold and dryness, and can persist unseen and unnoticed for months and years. Then when favourable conditions occur, they will germinate and grow into fresh colonies of the mould. Being so tiny, spores are carried over long distances – even across oceans – by the wind, which is the reason why most mould spores are found all over the world. Many of them do not germinate because the ambient conditions are not suitable, but there have been instances where growths of tropical moulds have occurred in cold countries where tropical conditions were maintained for industrial or research purposes.

One spore-forming mould is now known in the broad genus *Scopulariopsis*. About 28 different varieties have been recorded, one of these (probably the most important) being *Scopulariopsis brevicaulis*. During the nineteenth century it was given the name *Penicillium brevicaule* because of its apparent similarity to other organisms in the *Penicillium* genus. The word *brevicaule*, meaning 'short-stemmed', described the mould's appearance under the microscope. Later it was realised that the mould was not a *Penicillium* and in 1907 the biologist G. Bainier categorised the genus *Scopulariopsis*. At the same time he renamed *Penicillium brevicaule* (which had been identified by P. A. Saccardo in 1882) as *Scopulariopsis brevicaulis*.

Dissension and confusion about the name and the species persisted for some decades, but the name *Scopulariopsis* is now accepted, with *S. brevicaulis* being the most common organism in the genus.

S. brevicaulis is for the most part a totally harmless household organism. It grows on all kinds of decomposing organic matter and, unlike many moulds, flourishes on high-protein substances. Often it is found on mouldy cheese and in stale milk. There have been reports of human infection. Moulds of this genus have invaded open wounds, and attacked the feet of troops standing in waterlogged trenches during the First World War. It has been found in abscesses and ulcers, but such instances are rare in modern western societies.

Most mattresses become naturally infected by S. brevicaulis, particularly in those parts of the mattress which are warmed and where perspiration accumulates.

As mentioned in Chapter 3, following the deaths of many children in Italy, the possibility that they were caused by arsine poisoning was investigated by the Italian chemist, Gosio. His research showed that several moulds could liberate poisonous gas from arsenical pigments, one type being those of the genus Mucor, but by far the most important species was the mould then known as Penicillium brevicaule. He also demonstrated that the optimum conditions for production of the gas were the same as those which led to optimum growth of the mould. It was Gosio's opinion that the poisonous gas generated was not simply arsine but that other related arsenical gases were also present.

Clearly, Gosio was a very capable analytical chemist, because he also suggested that this reaction between compounds of arsenic and P. brevicaule would provide an extremely delicate test for the presence of arsenic in various materials. In those days very sensitive analysis was far more difficult than it is using modern electronic apparatus, and a technique capable of detecting arsenic to levels as low as one part per million was a useful addition to the science of analytical chemistry.

This type of reaction, involving the conversion of metals to gaseous compounds, is not unique. Although not known at the time when Gosio and Selmi made their discoveries, many such reactions are now recognised. An interesting example is the way in which mercury is converted into a poisonous gaseous compound (dimethylmercury), one of the reasons why the use of amalgam for filling teeth has become unpopular. Similar reactions occur with selenium and lead, again causing the production of very poisonous gases. But this knowledge was to come later.

The research into the formation of arsine, which began in the nineteenth century and continued for over 100 years, showed that the organism *S. brevicaulis* (in common with most strains of *Scopulariopsis*), was not always harmless. Under the right conditions – if there was even a trace of arsenic present where the mould was growing – this common household fungus could be deadly.

6

Enter Barry Richardson

One person who knew all about *Scopulariopsis brevicaulis* was Barry Richardson. His father had been a pharmaceutical chemist with an interest in wood preservation, so Barry grew up in a technical environment. English public school was followed by a degree in science from Southampton University, majoring in physiology and biochemistry. After graduating in 1960, Barry joined his father's chemical manufacturing business and at the same time carried out postgraduate research on wood preservation. In 1965 he commenced his own scientific consultancy.

It was a wide-ranging practice. He specialised in the deterioration and preservation of materials, especially building materials such as wood and stone, and related health matters. This led to the position of consultant to the Commonwealth War Graves Commission, the largest owner of commemorative stone in the world. His interest in structural materials culminated in the publication of a number of books on wood preservation which are regarded as definitive works in the field. He became deeply involved in marine biology, setting up a laboratory at St Peter Port on the island of Guernsey.

Barry's scientific achievements, which included the publication of over two hundred papers in scientific journals, led to his appointment as Chairman of the Association of Consulting Scientists and, in that capacity, to membership of the Parliamentary and Scientific Committee at Westminster.

By the time Peter Mitchell was grappling with his marquee problem, Barry Richardson had established his reputation as one of Britain's leading forensic scientists. Solving the marquee problem was simple; the cot death challenge raised by Peter Mitchell was a different proposition altogether.

Up to this point Barry hadn't given any particular thought to cot death. As in other countries where cot death was prevalent, it was seen as the preserve of medically trained people, and the opinions of non-medical persons were not welcome. So pervasive was the idea that cot death was a strictly medical matter that members of other disciplines almost ignored it. Of course, Barry was aware that Britain had a high cot death rate, which had been increasing for many years and was still rising, but publicity in Britain followed the line that cot death had many causes, all of them medical in one way or another.

Peter Mitchell's idea changed all that for Barry. Knowing, as a microbiologist, about *S. brevicaulis* and its propensity for generating arsine, and as a toxicologist about the intensely poisonous nature of this gas, he immediately realised that all the cot death factors which he had heard or read about fitted in with arsine poisoning.

Clearly, the first step was to investigate new cot mattresses. Peter Mitchell had been informed that the arsenical biocide OBPA was a regular addition to cot mattresses, so obviously this would be one avenue of testing. First, however, he would need to cultivate the fungus on the new mattresses. In his laboratory on Guernsey he already had a supply of *S. brevicaulis* – it was one of many cultures he routinely used in his research programmes – and he set about growing some of the fungus.

To do this, he put some of his *S. brevicaulis* culture onto a culture medium on which he knew the fungus would grow well. Tests like this are carried out in petri dishes, small glass or plastic dishes with loosely fitting covers. After a few days the fungus was growing vigorously.

Next he cut small pieces of the PVC plastic from the mattresses and placed them in the petri dishes, so that the fungus could grow on the plastic. Barry knew that if the fungus did grow it would consume some of the plasticiser in the plastic, and this would cause the plastic to shrink and wrinkle. Which is exactly what occurred.

Then it was a matter of testing for arsine. If there was any arsenic in the PVC mattress cover, the fungus – as well as consuming the plasticiser – would consume some of the OBPA which Barry expected to be present in the PVC.

Testing for arsine can be carried out in a number of ways. One is the method which was developed by a German chemist, Dr Gutzeit, in the early 1800s. Gutzeit's test, as it is called, depends on colour reactions in test papers. If the test papers change colour, this demonstrates the presence of arsine.

To Barry's surprise, there was no colour change, which meant that the PVC mattress covers apparently did not contain OBPA, or any other arsenical compound. Yet something strange did happen: Barry's assistant, Sue Kelly, said that whenever she worked on these petri dishes, she developed a headache. This was an almost certain indication of poisoning from some gas coming from the petri dishes. The question was: what was the gas? And why was it being formed?

Now was the time for some analytical chemistry. Barry's consulting chemist, Tim Cox, set about testing for arsenic in the PVC covers. He couldn't detect it, which led Barry, who was certain arsenic was there, to tease him about his competence (or lack of it). Tim replied that testing for minute amounts of arsenic was very difficult in the presence of so much antimony and phosphorus!

Tim's comment changed the whole focus. Barry knew that phosphorus would probably be present – PVC frequently contains phosphorus compounds – and that antimony was also likely. Then came a crucial lateral thought: nitrogen, phosphorus, arsenic and antimony are all members of Group Vb of the Periodic Table. He knew that S. brevicaulis could convert nitrogen to ammonia (NH_3) and arsenic to arsine (AsH_3). And since all four elements had very similar properties, could it be that S. brevicaulis would also convert phosphorus to phosphine (PH_3) and antimony to stibine (SbH_3)?

Barry knew that phosphine and stibine were, like arsine, very toxic gases – certainly toxic enough to give Sue Kelly a headache when she was working with the petri dishes. He consulted the chemical literature to see if there was any reference to the formation of these gases by the fungus, but did not find any. (Actually, there was a reference in an obscure journal but this did not come to light until some years later.)

Barry Richardson, however, is an experimenter. He immediately put his idea to the test, using the same petri dishes in which the fungus was growing on the PVC plastic, this time testing not for arsine but for phosphine and stibine. He soon found both of them.

Clearly, *S. brevicaulis could* cause the generation of phosphine from phosphorus compounds and stibine from antimony compounds.

Suddenly all the pieces of the jigsaw fell into place. If baby mattresses turned out to contain even one of the elements phosphorus, arsenic or antimony, and if *S. brevicaulis* (a very common fungus around the house) got into the mattress, there was a strong possibility that highly toxic gases would be generated – and these would certainly be capable of killing babies in a short space of time.

It was a fascinating thought.

And it fascinated Peter Mitchell. When Barry told him about the results obtained from new cot mattresses, Peter agreed straight away that it was now imperative to find mattresses on which babies had actually died of cot death and test these. Would these mattresses also show up the presence of the suspect elements? Would *S. brevicaulis* be found in them? And would the mattresses – or some of them – still be generating toxic gases?

The testing wouldn't be difficult; the hurdle was to get the mattresses. How was Peter going to locate families which had lost a baby, let alone persuade them to revisit their grief and hand over the mattress on which the baby had died (even assuming that the mattress had been kept)? In late 1988 he wrote to all the coroners in England and Wales to ask if they would co-operate. Many did, agreeing to release mattresses for testing. Hampshire and other police forces were generous in their support and over two hundred mattresses were eventually located. Peter arranged for these to be delivered to Barry for analysis at his Guernsey laboratory.

All of them would be tested: first for the fungus, to see if it was still in the mattress; and secondly, for the generation of one or more of the gases. If the second test was positive, it would prove that at least one of the suspect elements had been incorporated into the mattress during its manufacture.

Alongside this programme, used cot mattresses on which babies had *not* died would be tested, to find out whether these also were generating toxic gases.

The testing was completed by June 1989 and the results (several thousand of them after months of testing and re-testing) were nothing short of dramatic:

- Every mattress – whether a baby had died on it or not – was infected with S. *brevicaulis*, both the organism and its spores.

- As soon as the cot death mattresses were brought to blood heat, the fungus started growing again.

- All of the cot death mattresses contained one or more of the elements phosphorus, arsenic and antimony.

- Each cot death mattress started generating one or more of the gases phosphine, arsine and stibine after it had been brought to blood heat.

- Many of the non-cot death mattresses also generated phosphine, arsine or stibine, depending on the composition of the mattress materials.

The fungal growth was concentrated on the part of the mattress where the baby lay. This was not surprising, since the baby's perspiration, dribble, vomit and body heat would all cause the fungus to grow more readily.

And there was another telling observation. When *S. brevicaulis* grows, it frequently produces a pinkish stain, and such stains could be seen on some of the cot death mattresses in the shape of the baby where it had slept and then died. The presence of this pinkish stain was very interesting: the stain is the actual mould growing, and this fitted in with the Biblical reference in Leviticus 14 to a mould which was greenish or reddish. (See Chapter 3.)

Most cot mattresses in Britain are covered with PVC plastic but some (like New Zealand mattresses) are covered with fabric such as cotton and polyester. Modern 'vented' mattresses in both countries are covered only by netting, the mattress filling usually being some type of synthetic foam. Regardless of type, the fungus was found in *all* of the mattress coverings (whether plastic, fabric or netting), and in many of the foam mattress fillings. It was especially prevalent in foam which was covered only by netting. Clearly, therefore, toxic gases could be generated from *any* part of *any* mattress, provided it contained one of the suspect elements.

And if any of the mattresses generating stibine could be linked to excessive antimony present in the bodies of the babies' which had died on them, this would be compelling evidence of stibine poisoning. Barry managed to obtain six blood samples from such babies and he had these analysed for antimony by Dr Neil Ward at the Trace Element Laboratory, University of Surrey. The content of antimony in these blood samples was high (in one case eight times the normal level), establishing the link between the suspect mattresses and stibine poisoning.

When all the test results were put together, it was evident that most of the test mattress babies – whether they had lived or died – had been exposed to one or more of the gases. This was a sobering thought. It meant that many babies were being regularly exposed to toxic gases, and the outcome of that exposure depended only on how much of the toxic gas they inhaled. A sublethal dose would have no noticeable effect on a baby, but a higher concentration could kill it quickly.

Peter Mitchell was excited. He said to Barry, 'We'll crack this cot death problem in six months!' Barry, however, who had more experience of medical and scientific procrastination, replied, 'More like ten years!'

How right he was.

7

The Merry-Go-Round Begins

I t was never Barry Richardson's intention to become seriously involved in cot death research. Many organisations and individual researchers in Britain, including the high profile and well funded Foundation for the Study of Infant Deaths (FSID), were already looking at the problem. In any event, Barry had other demands on his time. But he realised that his discovery was important and that someone with the resources and ability to continue the research had to be told about it.

From early 1989 he had kept FSID informed of the progress of his investigations and in May 1989 addressed their Scientific Advisory Committee. FSID responded negatively: while agreeing that the hypothesis was consistent with other research findings, they decided that since it was 'unproven', there was no need for parents to take any action.

FSID did offer Barry a grant but he declined it. He didn't want to pursue the research, and thought that other researchers could do it better anyway. Nevertheless he was certainly keen for FSID to arrange further investigation of his hypothesis.

By this time Barry's study had advanced to the point where he had reported it to Members of Parliament in a briefing paper published by the Parliamentary Office for Science and Technology. Questions had been asked in the House of Commons. Barry had also submitted a preliminary paper to the *British Medical Journal*, hoping to encourage cot death researchers and pathologists to take his findings into account, but no response had been forthcoming from the *BMJ*.

Meanwhile, local radio and newspaper reporters had become intrigued by the fact that the police were delivering cot mattresses to Barry's premises. When they tracked him down for an explanation, he told them that he might have found a cause of cot death, but asked them – somewhat naively – to keep quiet until the research had been published in one of the medical journals.

The British news media aren't known for their reticence and it was soon clear that the embargo would not be respected. One morning in early June 1989, on arriving at the laboratory in Guernsey, Barry was surprised to find a television cameraman waiting for him, keen to take photos of the laboratory in preparation for a television interview. Barry was in the process of explaining to the cameraman that he was not aware of any interview, when the phone rang. It was the television producer, requesting an immediate interview because the news services were already carrying reports that he had discovered the cause of cot death. The news spread like wildfire. Within 24 hours, the Guernsey laboratory was besieged by newspaper, radio and television reporters.

It was a great opportunity. Barry wanted to get his message across that poisoning by the toxic gases could easily be avoided: either buy a new mattress for the baby, or cover its mattress with polythene sheeting. The media responded in fine style and Barry's recommendation was spread immediately throughout the length and breadth of Britain.

Several medical researchers responded in a rather different manner: Barry Richardson was only a materials scientist, so what did he know about cot death?

The *BMJ*, clearly miffed, rejected Barry's paper on the ground of prior publicity. (Actually, the *BMJ* had been sitting on the paper for months, despite Barry's warning that they were taking too long to assess it and the story was about to break.)

But other people *were* listening. Parents who previously were content to re-use cot mattresses from one baby to the next started buying new ones, to the extent that sales of new mattresses jumped by 15%. A number of cot mattress manufacturers sidled up to Barry to ask him whether their mattresses were safe, and if not, what they should do. More importantly, after rising for the previous 30 years, the cot death rate in Britain immediately tumbled, on a downward trend which continued for the next four years.

Despite their scepticism, FSID were sufficiently motivated to commission the first outside scientific investigation into Barry's research. In 1990 they arranged for Dr Colin Simpson and Dr Anne Donovan at the University of London to analyse nine PVC cot mattress covers used by cot death babies. Their task was to analyse the covers for arsenic and antimony, and to attempt to generate toxic gases from the covers.

Drs Donovan and Simpson found high levels of antimony in five of the nine mattress covers and trace amounts in the other four but they were not able to generate stibine from the covers. FSID duly reported that their research did not confirm Barry Richardson's conclusion that toxic gases could be given off from cot mattresses.

The reasons for the failure to detect the toxic gases were not apparent at the time but are now understood: see Chapter 12. Others were to make the same mistakes.

Needless to say, throughout this time the indefatigable Peter Mitchell had not been idle. Starting with his local MP, he set in train a massive letter-writing campaign, bombarding with information anyone who could help publicise the hypothesis: Ministers of the Crown, Members of Parliament, Government departments, coroners, doctors and the news media. As early as January 1989 he and Barry had written to the Department of Health, suggesting that arsine from cot mattresses might be implicated in cot deaths.

The Department had replied that in their opinion the idea had no credibility, but a visit in March 1990 by Peter and Barry to Chief Medical Officer Sir Donald Acheson had led to a positive result. Acheson recognised that the Richardson hypothesis represented a major challenge to conventional medical thinking on cot death and he was sufficiently impressed by the research to set up in March 1990 a group of independent experts to investigate it.

The Turner Committee, as it came to be known, included several professors of medicine, professors of chemistry and biology, a consultant in paediatric pathology and a poisons expert. They were assisted by a number of highly qualified officials from various Government departments. The chairman was Professor Paul Turner, Professor of Clinical Pharmacology at St Bartholomew's Medical College, London, and chairman of the Government's advisory committee on toxicity.

The Turner Committee, which was to spend more than a quarter of a million pounds on its task, began investigations in April 1990. Experimental work was carried out at the Laboratory of the Government Chemist and the International Mycological Institute and the Committee duly published its Report in June 1991. According to the Report, the Richardson hypothesis could not be confirmed, because the generation of phosphine, arsine and stibine by *Scopulariopsis brevicaulis* could not be replicated.

In fact, this was not true. The chemists who had the task of replicating Barry Richardson's results did succeed in generating toxic gas from arsenic and antimony but not from phosphorus. But the positive result from antimony was ignored by the Committee as being due to contamination. They had carried out many tests which gave negative results and based their Report on those results only.

In a scientific examination any anomalous result must be clarified. Even though the weight of evidence may appear to be against a rogue result, that result must be explained before it can be ignored. If it cannot be explained, research must continue (perhaps by modified methods) until it can be explained. When reporting scientific conclusions, there is no place for a finding based on a 'majority of results'.

The Turner Committee, however, based its Report on just such a majority of results decision. In fact, the results had *confirmed* the Richardson hypothesis, albeit not consistently.

(Although not apparent at the time, it is now clear why the Turner Committee were unable to generate the gases consistently, even on their own 'spiked' samples. This issue is dealt with in the technical discussion in Chapter 12.)

The Turner Report was a mixed document. Instead of trying to resolve the anomalies and find out why the gas results had been inconsistent, the Committee simply walked away from the question and deferred it.

Sir Donald Acheson's stance was also equivocal. When setting up the Turner Committee in March 1990 he had commented that he didn't believe that mattresses were involved in cot deaths; but now, when asked by a reporter at the launch of the Report whether a new mattress for each baby was a good idea, he agreed that it was.

And the Report of the Turner Committee was also equivocal: it contained a recommendation that if antimony fire retardant was used in mattresses, the levels of arsenic in the antimony should be as low as possible – a tacit admission that mattresses could generate arsine. It even went so far as to question the safety of plasticisers and fire retardants themselves, given the potential toxicity of these materials and their *foreseeable breakdown products* – another tacit admission that chemicals added to mattresses could generate toxic gases.

A further problem flawed the Report of the Turner Committee. Its terms of reference were very restrictive and didn't allow for any tests on post-mortem samples of blood and body tissue of cot death babies.

As previously mentioned, Barry Richardson had commissioned analyses of blood taken from six cot death babies whose mattresses had been found to contain antimony. These blood analyses had revealed high antimony levels, consistent with poisoning by stibine and confirming the Richardson hypothesis.

Barry had published these findings before the Turner Committee wrote their Report but the Committee chose not to investigate this aspect of his work. Admittedly, testing post-mortem samples was not specifically mentioned in the terms of reference but that was really no impediment; the Committee certainly had the power and the facilities to obtain and analyse post-mortem samples. Having erroneously concluded that antimony was not a problem, they took the matter no further.

A significant opportunity had been lost. Professor West, Emeritus Professor of Analytical Chemistry at the University of Aberdeen and a member of the Turner Committee, later came round to this way of thinking and in a television interview in November 1994 agreed that post-mortem samples should have been analysed and expressed his regret that this wasn't done.

To the credit of the Turner Committee, they did make two useful recommendations: that the Government should put in place a British Standard for the resistance of cot mattresses to the growth of certain micro-organisms; and that fungi found on the mattresses of cot death babies should be specifically investigated. (These recommendations were ignored by the Department of Health.)

As Professor Derek Bryce-Smith (a leading campaigner against lead in petrol) stated in 1994:

> The kindest thing I can say about [the Turner Report] is that it was really rather inadequate. It certainly is not the last word on the subject. We want more work carried out by other people who are at arm's length from political or industrial pressure.

It is interesting to speculate why the Turner Report was incomplete and even contained internal contradictions. At the outset Sir Donald Acheson expected the Committee to report within three months, but in the event it took fifteen. So many observers and consultants were co-opted that they eventually outnumbered the original seven Committee members. Rumours emerged that there was strong disagreement within the group, leading to the 'safety net' sentences in the final Report.

Certainly the Committee believed that there were many

causes of cot death – the conventional view at the time – but their reluctance to accept the gas poisoning hypothesis may have been due to more immediate considerations. Fire retardants had been made mandatory for cot mattresses – against the wishes of manufacturers – and it would have been politically embarrassing to have to admit now, after repeated warnings from Barry Richardson, that retardants might have led to cot deaths. Not only that, but the Government had already been recommended to test blood of cot death babies for antimony, which would have revealed evidence of stibine poisoning, and they had failed to take this advice. Pathologists and coroners around the country had also ignored the advice. Furthermore, cot mattress manufacturers, who had been aware of Richardson's work since June 1989, were at risk from damages claims if the Turner Committee endorsed his findings.

Whatever the explanation, the June 1991 publication of the Turner Report officially stonewalled the Richardson hypothesis. According to the Department of Health, the theory had no validity. The news media flagged it away and FSID kept on denouncing it. In the words of FSID Secretary-General Dr Joyce Epstein: 'I hope this puts an end to scare stories about toxic gases.'

Interestingly, however, and to the relief of parents, the cot death rate throughout Britain continued to fall. It had peaked in 1986–1988, but following Barry's publicity in June 1989, the rate for England and Wales had come down by 38%, from 2.30 per 1000 live births in 1988 to only 1.44 in 1991.

It would later be claimed by FSID and the British Department of Health that this dramatic reduction in cot death was due to their adoption of what was subsequently called 'Back to Sleep' (the recommendation that babies be put down to sleep on their backs rather than on their sides or face down). But at the time of the Turner Report, face-up sleeping was contrary to official Department of Health policy. The 'Back to Sleep' campaign was not officially launched until December 1991.

As shown in the graph on p. 56, there was only one reason for this fall in the British cot death rate: the publication of the

Richardson hypothesis. Officialdom may not have wanted to listen, but mattress manufacturers did, and in some cases removed antimony from their products. Parents listened as well. Many bought new mattresses, while others wrapped existing mattresses in polythene.

Even in the face of the consistently falling cot death rate, officialdom in Britain procrastinated. Confusion was evident in an August 1992 letter from the Secretary of State for Health:

> Mr Richardson is the only person to have detected any toxic gases produced by fungal action from cot mattresses.
> *(Actually the Turner Committee had done so as well. They detected stibine and arsine generated from a mattress.)*

> Blood tests for potentially toxic substances are of value only if a normal level has been established.
> *(This ignores the fact that stibine, the toxic substance in question, is decomposed in the body within minutes of ingestion.)*

> There is no established normal level of blood antimony for infants.
> *(The normal range for antimony in infant blood had, in fact, been established.)*

> What is clear is that there are no reports of symptoms indicative of antimony poisoning from the post-mortems on [cot death] cases.
> *(Of course not: the toxic substance was stibine, not antimony.)*

Uninformed thinking of this type has clouded the cot death debate for years.

Research scientist Barry responded predictably to the Turner Committee findings. In July 1990 he presented a paper to a joint meeting of the British Society for Allergy and Environmental Medicine (BSAEM) and the American Academy of Environmental Medicine. He also continued writing: in 1991 papers and

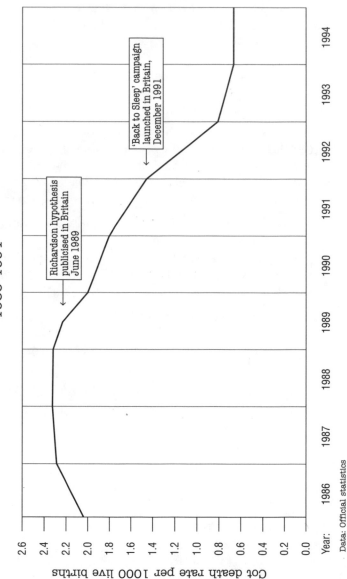

COT DEATH RATES IN BRITAIN:
1986–1994

Richardson hypothesis
publicised in Britain
June 1989

'Back to Sleep' campaign
launched in Britain,
December 1991

Cot death rate per 1000 live births

Year:

Data: Official statistics

COT DEATH RATES IN BRITAIN:
1986–1994

The dramatic reduction in the British cot death rate brought about by the June 1989 announcement of the Richardson hypothesis is unmistakeable.

The British Department of Health 'Back to Sleep' campaign was officially launched in December 1991.

This graph refutes the later claim made by the Department of Health, FSID and others that 'Back to Sleep' accounted for the 73% reduction in the cot death rate over the period 1989–1993.

'Back to Sleep' was responsible for about half the reduction in the cot death rate during the 1992 year. Richardson's publicity had resulted in the rate falling 38% by December 1991. During the 1992 year the rate fell by 46%, of which 'Back to Sleep' was responsible for about 23 percentage points and Richardson's publicity for about 23 percentage points.

Put another way, of the total fall in the cot death rate of 1.54/1000 from 2.31 in 1986–1988 to 0.77 in 1992, 'Back to Sleep' was responsible for about 0.34 deaths/1000 births and Richardson's publicity for the remaining 1.2/1000. Any other interpretation of the statistics ignores the facts.

Note that the rate levelled off during 1993 and 1994. It appears to be continuing at about the 1994 rate. This is due to the presence of phosphorus in mattress materials. Face-up sleeping is not very effective against phosphine because this gas has a relatively low vapour density.

Further reduction in the British cot death rate cannot be expected until new mattresses are free from phosphorus as well as antimony, and all parents using older mattresses cover them with polythene, or some other gas-impermeable sheeting known to be free from the harmful elements.

letters were published in the *Journal of Clinical Ecology*, *The Lancet*, and *Complementary Medical Research*.

But if he was going to embark on a substantial piece of literature research and writing, Barry needed funding. He had already spent over £100,000 of his own money on laboratory research, to say nothing of the services provided free of charge by his staff. His business was suffering.

Furthermore the message wasn't getting through as well as he wanted. Technical papers just didn't reach the right audience. Barry realised the need existed for a book which would give the whole picture – the history of cot death, research, results, conclusions and bibliography – but he couldn't afford the time or the money to do it. Then in July 1991 there was a breakthrough.

Tomy UK Ltd, a Japanese manufacturer and major British supplier of toys and nursery items, had been following the news of Barry's work. Recognising what Barry had already achieved and concerned at the slow progress towards acceptance of his findings in relation to cot mattress materials, they offered him sponsorship for the next stage of his research programme.

Tomy were thinking in terms of more laboratory work but Barry explained that he had completed his experiments in the summer of 1990. The need now was for a comprehensive review of cot death reports to see how they related to his findings. Tomy agreed, and provided a grant to enable him to concentrate on the project.

The result was a 60-page book entitled *Cot Death: Must Babies Still Die?* launched at a press conference held at St Bartholomew's Hospital in November 1991. It had taken three months to write, and brought together – in a form that the general public could understand – epidemiology on the one hand and science on the other. A massive amount of previous cot death literature was drawn upon (240 published papers and books appear in the bibliography) and the epidemiological observations about cot death were linked up with the chemical findings.

Copies had been sent to the Secretary of State for Health and to the Turner Committee.

The book answered questions which had never been answered before, such as 'Why is sleeping position important?' 'Why does overheating increase cot death?' 'Why does aspirin appear to cause cot death?' 'Why do babies with minor illnesses appear to be more at risk?' and 'Why don't babies less than one month old die of cot death?'

Its conclusion was inescapable: cot death was due to poisoning.

Using the research which had been carried out in Guernsey, and drawing on his own extensive knowledge of the dangerous properties of *S. brevicaulis*, Barry reaffirmed his conviction that poisonous gases generated in cot mattresses were killing babies.

And more than that: Barry was convinced that this was the *prime* cause of cot death, perhaps the *only* cause. Plenty of people had consistently observed the same features of cot death, and many of these features had been pounced on in isolation as the cause of cot death. But it was clear to Barry that these observations – all of them true – were still only observations. They were 'symptoms' rather than causes, statistics rather than an explanation. But Barry had discovered an answer which tallied with all of them and fitted them all together – without a single discrepancy.

Citing the Turner Report, which had been published only a few months before, Barry pointed out its shortcomings and limitations and explained why the Committee had reached its erroneous conclusion. He protested:

It is not surprising that the group reported that the hypothesis was unproven through lack of any independent supporting data, as the group ignored any data and avoided any investigations that might have confirmed the hypothesis.

However, as Barry realised, the Turner Committee hadn't actually made up their minds about gas generation. They had left the door open. As he put it:

The group recommended that the potential toxicity of additives in mattress materials and their breakdown products should be investigated, emphasising the possible significance of arsenic contamination of the antimony trioxide which is used as a fire retardant additive and the risk of formation of *toxic volatile compounds*. The group recommended that the hazards associated with *microbial contamination* should also be investigated.

So ended Barry's commentary on the Turner Committee; but these niceties cut no ice with the news media or the cot death establishment. The latter had been delighted with what they saw as short shrift given to the hypothesis by the Turner Committee, being sure that it had been effectively disposed of. However, the November 1991 publication of the Tomy report again drew public attention to Barry's work, and relations between FSID and Barry deteriorated. In December 1991 Joyce Epstein, FSID Secretary-General, wrote a stinging letter to the press:

> Mr Richardson claims he has 'new' evidence; he has not. What Mr Richardson does have is new financial backing – from a non-medical source – which enables him to buy the services of an excellent publicity agent. It is a great shame that Mr Richardson's unsubstantiated claims continue to add needlessly to parental anxiety about cot death.

Strong words about the person who had achieved the first reduction ever in cot death in Britain, especially when he had spent £100,000 of his own money on cot death research. And the £5000 received from Tomy – far from recompensing the three months' research – had scarcely covered the cost of publishing and distributing the resulting book. Coming from the handsomely funded FSID, it was a bit rich.

While Barry's work and its publication had led to the first fall in the British cot death rate in decades, researchers in other countries had noted a connection between face-down sleeping and an increased risk of cot death. From the mid-1980s onwards the idea that sleeping position might be a cot death risk factor had been raised in countries such as Ireland, France, the Netherlands and Australia, but when first proposed, it was met with forceful opposition from some quarters.

By 1991 the opposition had been largely stilled (though not in Britain). The New Zealand Cot Death Study, a wide-ranging three-year investigation into the epidemiology of cot death, had shown once and for all that babies sleeping face up were less likely to die of cot death, though no explanation for the finding had been advanced.

In Britain Barry Richardson had been advocating face-up sleeping since 1989 but the benefit of this practice had been denied by the British Department of Health and FSID. As late as August 1991 Baroness Hooper, Parliamentary Undersecretary for Health, was still denying that face-up sleeping could be advantageous. But on 31 October 1991, faced with overwhelming evidence and under heavy media pressure, the Department reversed their policy and endorsed face-up sleeping. On 10 December the Secretary of State for Health officially launched the £2,000,000 'Back to Sleep' campaign. It quickly caught on with the British public and the cot death rate continued to fall, indeed at a greater rate. Yet it was evident from the pleasing statistics for the previous 2 1/2 years that sleeping position was far from the total answer.

Away from the limelight, Peter Mitchell had been methodically working his way through the mountain of data which he had accumulated on cot death. Much of it seemed anecdotal and unrelated, but he was about to recognise a piece of epidemiology which turned out to be probably the most important observation ever about cot death.

Peter had pestered the Department of Statistics for all their facts and figures about cot death: when babies died, and which babies died, and where they died, and how many died, and so on. The data poured in and laboriously he set about analysing it – all by hand, because computers aren't his forte.

Out of this came a fundamental observation: that the rate of cot death doubled from the first baby in a family to the second; and doubled again from the second to the third; and increased from the third to the fourth. Babies of unmarried mothers were more than six times more likely to die of cot death than the first babies of married mothers.

He graphed this data. It showed, once and for all, that the conventional explanations and theories and so-called risk factors for cot death – like smoking, face-up sleeping, not breastfeeding, and overheating – were no more than incidentals, smokescreens for the real cause. If any of these factors were the ultimate cause of cot death, how could it be explained that the third baby in a family, for example, was at far greater risk than the first? Or that the babies of unmarried mothers were six times more at risk? Other researchers had previously noted these statistics but had apparently not appreciated their significance.

Peter already knew that cot deaths often occurred on used mattresses – of the 200 cot death mattresses he collected for Barry, about 95% had been previously used by other infants – but surely it was not being suggested that mothers were changing . their babycare methods from one baby to the next? For example, with all the publicity promoting face-up sleeping, was it credible that mothers who had put their first babies to sleep face up were putting their later babies to sleep face down? Obviously not.

Yet if face-up sleeping was succeeding with the first baby, why wasn't it succeeding as well with second and third babies? Or with babies of unmarried mothers?

Again, if lack of smoking around the baby was succeeding with the first baby, why wasn't it succeeding so well in the case of subsequent babies? And likewise breastfeeding? Or avoiding overheating?

The answer was apparent: all these were just risk factors, 'symptoms', observed features which ran parallel with cot death but which didn't account for it.

The unexpected finding that the cot death rate rose among later births demanded an explanation. The traditional cot death theories failed to tally with it, but the Richardson hypothesis fitted it exactly. Parents pass mattresses down from one child to the next. The first baby in a family is likely to have a brand new mattress, but this mattress is often re-used for the second arrival, and maybe the third. If the mother is unmarried (which frequently equates with being poorer), the likelihood becomes very high that she will borrow a mattress or buy a second-hand one.

The longer a cot mattress is used, the better established becomes the fungus. There is more of it, and it is also more active. Therefore, if any of the dangerous elements are present in the mattress, more gas is generated. It's as simple as that.

The answer to one known factor about cot death became clear immediately: why babies under one month old seldom succumb. Even with a used mattress, it takes a while after a baby has started sleeping on it regularly for the fungus in the mattress to develop.

Here, then, in Peter Mitchell's finding of rising cot death rate among later births, lay the fundamental statistic about cot death, against which any proposition on cot death must be tested: the ultimate piece of epidemiology. In early 1995 I reproduced Peter Mitchell's hand-drawn graph of the finding in computer-generated form. This is shown on page 64.

Peter kept up-to-date his statistics on the rising cot death rate among later births, and the same finding was repeated in 1993 and 1994.

The significance of the graph is perhaps not apparent at first sight but it portrays an undeniable and repeated statistic. Any proposition regarding the cause of cot death – and there have been more than two hundred – is worthless unless it checks with this graph. Any suggested cause which is compatible with this graph is worthy of consideration but all ideas which are incompatible with it must be discarded.

The traditional epidemiologists may have noticed this trend of rising cot death rate among later births. In fact, some figures confirming it appeared in the New Zealand Cot

COT DEATH RATES FOR FIRST AND LATER BABIES AND BABIES OF UNMARRIED MOTHERS: BRITAIN, 1992

THE COT DEATH COVER-UP?

Cot death rate per 1000 live births

First babies of wealthy parents
All first babies
Second babies
Third babies
Fourth and later babies
Babies of unmarried mothers

Data: Official statistics

COT DEATH RATES FOR FIRST AND LATER BABIES AND BABIES OF UNMARRIED MOTHERS: BRITAIN, 1992

This graph, developed originally by Peter Mitchell, is arguably the most important piece of epidemiology relating to the cause of cot death. The range of cot death risk from the lowest group (first babies of wealthy parents) to the highest group (babies of unmarried mothers) is 1:22.

This data is part of the overwhelming proof that there is only one cause of cot death and destroys any argument that cot death has a medical cause.

It demonstrates that the more times a mattress is used from one baby to the next, the greater is the risk of cot death.

This accounts for the higher cot death rates in less well-off families, who are more likely to use second-hand mattresses. If a mattress contains the dangerous elements, and the fungus has become established in the mattress during prior use, the output of toxic gas commences sooner and is greater in volume.

Death Study but without any comment from the authors.

The data was all there in British Government statistics, unnoticed and unremarked on by the highly paid researchers. It was Peter Mitchell, a businessman with no medical, scientific or academic background, who finally realised what it meant.

8

Interlude

U p to the end of 1991 I had never heard of Peter Mitchell, or Barry Richardson and his hypothesis, or the Turner Committee. After the study in Southland was completed, I returned to Canada, where my wife and I had emigrated.

Of course, the cot death situation in Canada was of interest to me. News items appeared from time to time, drawing attention to the high cot death rate in British Columbia and Alberta and to the fact that no solution appeared to be in sight. I kept writing to newspapers and people quoted in the press, reiterating my conviction that cot death (known in the USA and Canada as 'crib death') was due to environmental poisoning. I also bombarded doctors and cot death societies in a number of countries with information on my proposition, but the concept never elicited any response.

I kept up my correspondence with Peter Muller at the *Southland Times* until he retired from his position as editor. Since publication of the Southland study Peter had sent me the Southland cot death statistics as he received them month by month. The rate stayed at a low level, still well below the rest of New Zealand.

Peter obtained these statistics from the Southland Area Health Board. As editor of the local newspaper he enjoyed access to this sort of information, but when he retired the flow of data came to an abrupt halt. I wrote to the new editor of the *Southland Times*, asking if he was interested in continuing the Southland study, but there was no response. Likewise, no response was forthcoming from the Southland Area Health Board when I wrote to them for statistics. Peter Muller told me later the reason for the Health Board's decision: I was not 'a recognised cot death researcher'.

It seemed as though progress in New Zealand had reached a stalemate, when late in 1991 news of the Richardson hypothesis reached New Zealand. On 30 November the *New Zealand Herald* carried an article setting out the main points of the hypothesis: that materials used in cot mattresses were the prime cause of cot death, generating volatile and deadly gaseous compounds from phosphorus, arsenic and antimony.

According to the article, the hypothesis lined up with the results of the New Zealand Cot Death Study regarding the dangers of face-down sleeping and overwrapping babies in cots. It also explained why the use of sheepfleeces in Australia and New Zealand had been a contributing factor to cot death: the answer lay in the presence of phosphorus, arsenic and antimony in fleeces.

When I received a copy of this article in Canada, I was thrilled. Having believed since 1986 that babies were being poisoned by toxic gases generated by microbiological activity on something in their cots, I now had the answer to the question which had baffled me for five years: the identity of the poisonous gases. They were phosphine, arsine and stibine and/or closely related compounds.

Others were not so thrilled. The cot death division of the National Child Health Research Foundation shot back a reaction immediately. According to Dr Shirley Tonkin, the division co-ordinator, many upset parents had called her since the *Herald* report had appeared and her response was quite clear. New Zealanders should ignore the hypothesis, she said. Barry Richardson had an idea, but no proof at all, and parents need not worry about it.

It would be interesting to know whether Shirley Tonkin had actually studied any of Barry's written material on the topic. No-one reading this could possibly jump to the conclusion that he had no proof at all.

Obviously I had to find Barry Richardson, so starting with my photocopy of the *Herald* report I set about tracking him down. According to the *Herald*, he was 'a Guernsey-based research biochemist and physiologist'. I had visited Jersey in the past but had never been to Guernsey. I knew that the main town on the island was St Peter Port, so the first step was to write to the postmaster there, enclosing a letter to the person who was researching cot death. Within days I received a letter back from Barry. It was a lengthy response from one scientist to another, detailing the hypothesis and expressing interest in my Southland work. One cogent paragraph showed that Barry was evidently accustomed to stonewalling from the cot death establishment.

Expressing his hope that he and I did not suffer from 'the tunnel vision that seems to affect medical researchers', Barry was obviously as keen as I was to keep in contact.

I read his publication *Cot Death: Must Babies Still Die?* with avid interest. It detailed his research and stated:

> It must be concluded that the primary cause of [cot death] is generation of phosphine, arsine, stibine and related toxic gases through biodeterioration of mattress materials containing phosphorus, arsenic and antimony compounds . . .
> The prone sleeping position is a contributory factor in [cot death] and avoidance will reduce but not eliminate the risk; the [cot death] risk will only be eliminated or reduced to the insignificant level experienced in unaffected countries such as Japan by avoiding the primary cause which is the presence of phosphorus, arsenic and antimony compounds in cot mattress materials.

Armed now with detailed scientific support for my original proposition and knowing the identity of the toxic gases and how they were formed, I renewed my worldwide letter-writing campaign.

Barry kept up his campaign too, focusing on the technical journals. Despite all the criticism and opposition, some people had taken notice of Barry's cot death research and by now he had been appointed Honorary Research Fellow at King Alfred's College in Winchester in recognition of this work. In February 1993 he presented a paper which was published in 1994 in the *Journal of the Forensic Science Society*. It was entitled 'Sudden Infant Death Syndrome: a possible primary cause'.

But the cot death establishment paid little attention, and there the matter sat.

9

The Television Producer

At 2 am on a Friday morning in November 1994 the phone rang. Joan Shenton, a television producer based in London, was on the line and wanted to talk about Barry Richardson's hypothesis.

Joan, a freelancer with her own production company, Meditel Productions, specialises in documentaries on medicine-related topics. With over twenty years' experience in the field, she has gained a reputation for well researched, hard-hitting stories. Reading between the lines of the cot death news reports which appeared from time to time in Britain, she had realised in 1993 that something was going on. And she suspected there was a story in it.

Making television documentaries is all about contacting the right people and asking the right questions. Joan knew that if she was to produce a marketable programme on such a sensitive and technical topic as cot death, the research would have to be meticulous. In September 1993 she got in touch with Barry Richardson.

This came as a complete surprise to Barry, who of course was only too delighted to impart everything he had discovered about cot death.

He also passed on correspondence between himself and the Foundation for the Study of Infant Death (FSID), letters which made Joan suspicious. A typical exchange between FSID and Barry led him to warn them in December 1991:

I must ask you to ensure that your Foundation representatives do not make any statements, either verbally or in writing, which are incorrect or untruthful in relation to my involvement in SIDS research . . .

I am often asked, both by the media and by other researchers, whether I can explain why your Foundation is so vociferous in its attempts to discredit my research instead of accepting it as just another contribution to knowledge of SIDS.

Coming from mild-mannered, academically inclined research scientist Barry Richardson, these were strong words. What prompted them, Joan wondered.

She got in touch with FSID, who appeared to be very concerned about the hypothesis being aired on television.

Pursuing her enquiries, she came upon Professor Jack Pridham, Professor of Biochemistry at Royal Holloway College at the University of London. And here the feedback was strikingly different. Pridham had been quietly carrying out his own experiments to test Barry's hypothesis, with his students participating. He believed it was possible that gases were being produced from cot mattress chemicals and felt that the debate on Barry's hypothesis should be re-opened.

By the time Joan had wrapped up her investigation, she and her assistant, Roger Lavender, had been in contact with researchers, cot death society officers, several Members of Parliament, public servants, academics (including Professor Paul Turner of the Turner Committee), medical experts, doctors, mattress manufacturers and retailers – and, of course, bereaved parents.

And she had concluded that she was onto something.

Among Joan's interviewees was Mr John Watt, Chairman of the Association of Consulting Scientists and a blood specialist. He pointed to flaws in the Turner Committee's research methods. It seemed questionable whether the Turner Committee had got it right.

The script for Joan's programme made riveting reading, but the established television companies were sceptical and unimpressed. Eighteen months later Joan was still hawking it round the industry, trying to interest a buyer.

The *Cook Report*, produced by Central Television (now Carlton Television) in Birmingham, had been making hard-hitting consumer affairs television programmes for about ten years. By now it was a virtual institution but that fact had not softened its incisive approach. New Zealand-born anchorman Roger Cook pursued his stories with fearless determination. Programmes were broadcast weekly, achieving massive viewer ratings.

When Joan Shenton turned up at the studio in Birmingham with her story, Roger and his producer, Peter Salkeld, recognised it as classic *Cook Report* and decided to give it a go, with Joan participating as co-producer.

Obviously, the topic of cot death – which had been the subject of so much speculation – could be approached in many ways, but a 23-minute television documentary calls for a sharp focus. Roger and Peter were convinced by the Richardson hypothesis and its ramifications, but even the hypothesis would have to be narrowed down to its salient point. Barry told Joan: concentrate on the generation of stibine from new and used cot mattresses, and the detection of antimony in body samples taken from cot death babies; while you're doing this, try to obtain body samples from babies which have died from other causes; and phone Jim Sprott, because he identified the mechanism of cot death years ago and understands the hypothesis.

By this time my wife and I had returned to live in New Zealand and had re-established ourselves in Auckland. When Joan phoned in early November 1994, it was to ask me to provide a telephone interview for the *Cook Report* programme to be screened on 17 November. The programme was to be called 'The Cot Death Poisonings' and its aim was to explain the Richardson hypothesis. She would have preferred a studio interview in Birmingham, but apologized that the programme budget did not run to the cost of an airfare from New Zealand to Britain.

The *Cook Report* had taken Barry's advice. Having obtained a supply of new and used cot mattresses, they had these analysed for phosphorus, arsenic and antimony. As expected, phosphorus and antimony – sometimes one element and sometimes both – were present in both new and used mattresses, frequently at high concentrations.

They followed this up with tests for stibine generation using *Scopulariopsis brevicaulis*. Barry Richardson grew cultures on the mattress samples and absorbed the generated gas onto his usual test papers. Public analyst Ron Rooney then analysed the test papers and detected the presence of antimony, confirming that stibine had been generated from the mattresses.

Obtaining post-mortem samples taken from cot death and other babies hadn't been so simple. Over the years many thousands of samples had been taken by pathologists and some were still being held by hospitals. But getting samples released for analysis was quite another matter. Even if parents agreed, the consent of the hospital and the coroner was required. It looked like a ponderous and time-consuming prospect, when suddenly there was a breakthrough: Sheffield Children's Hospital agreed to co-operate. The hospital had meticulously kept body samples taken from both cot death and non-cot death babies in the hope that one day these might assist in research, and it provided the *Cook Report* with a large number of samples. A few additional samples were also obtained from nearby hospitals.

It is known that if antimony is ingested into the body as a result of chronic (continuing or long-term) exposure, it accumulates predominantly in the liver, kidneys and hair. Consequently liver samples (the tissue samples usually taken from cot death babies) give a very reliable indication of past exposure to antimony.

Fifty-five liver samples – 40 taken from cot death babies and 15 from non-cot death babies – were analysed for antimony by Dr Andrew Taylor of the Robens Institute Trace Element Laboratory at the University of Surrey. The analytical results were staggering: of the samples from non-cot death babies, 14 did not contain any measurable antimony and one contained a small amount; whereas of the 40 samples from cot death babies, 20 contained significant levels of antimony (15 at high levels).

At the same time, Dr Taylor analysed 52 samples of blood from the same group of babies. Antimony was found in 19 of 39 cot death babies and 2 of 13 non-cot death babies, but these results did not always correlate with the liver result for the same baby.

On the face of it, this may appear to weaken the impact of the liver results, but actually it doesn't. Rather, it confirms something else known about antimony poisoning: that acute poisoning (poisoning at the time of death) shows up especially in the blood and lungs, even though it may not show up in the liver. (Interestingly, recent research in the USA has identified high antimony levels in lung tissue taken from cot death babies.)

Put together, Dr Taylor's liver and serum results showed that two-thirds of the cot death babies had been exposed to antimony.

Joan Shenton and Peter Salkeld set about filming their programme, using the liver results to demonstrate that the Richardson hypothesis should be taken seriously. The programme was almost wrapped up, when they found a useful ally: television presenter Anne Diamond.

Successful television personalities in Britain enjoy a huge following among the public. Even in a country of over 60 million people they are household names. Presenter Anne Diamond – aged 40, glamorous and eloquent – had this status. But she and her television producer husband, Mike Hollingsworth, had suffered the grief of a cot death. Their third child, Sebastian, had died in July 1991 at the age of four months.

In the aftermath of this loss Anne had become a cot death activist. Her name was associated with an appeal launched by the *Sun* newspaper which raised £200,000 for cot death research. Having heard about the New Zealand Cot Death Study, and especially the success being achieved by face-up sleeping, she decided to go to New Zealand and see for herself. She returned to Britain totally convinced and took part in a Thames Television

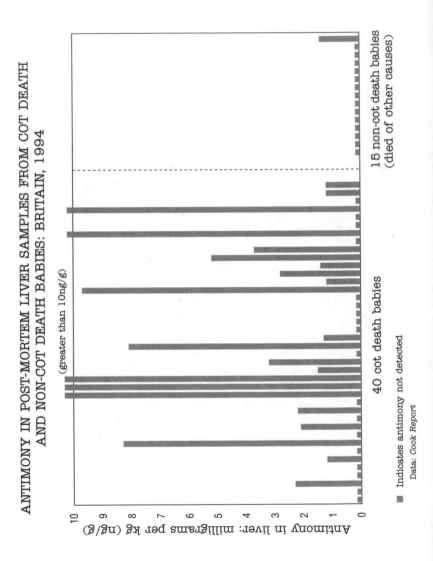

ANTIMONY IN POST-MORTEM LIVER SAMPLES FROM COT DEATH AND NON-COT DEATH BABIES: BRITAIN, 1994

Data: *Cook Report*

ANTIMONY IN POST-MORTEM LIVER SAMPLES FROM COT DEATH AND NON-COT DEATH BABIES: BRITAIN, 1994

This graph depicts the results of analysis of post-mortem liver samples, 40 from babies which died of cot death and 15 from babies which died of other known causes. The only feasible source of the elevated amounts of antimony in the samples is from stibine generated from the babies' mattresses.

The much greater incidence of antimony in the livers of the cot death babies is very apparent. The one baby in the non-cot death group with a positive antimony result had apparently been exposed to stibine before it died of some other cause.

Of the elements phosphorus, arsenic and antimony, only antimony can be tracked meaningfully in the bodies of cot death victims. Exposure to phosphine and arsine cannot be detected in this manner because of the significant amounts of phosphorus and arsenic (especially phosphorus) naturally present in the body.

This Week programme on cot death. This programme was about
to go to air on 31 October 1991, when the Department of Health
announced their new policy on face-up sleeping.

The upper echelons of television are a small world, so Roger
Cook knew Anne well and was aware of her background in cot
death. Could her involvement help publicise the hypothesis, he
wondered. Roger now firmly believed that Richardson was
correct and it had become more than just another programme.
Lives were at stake.

And then he thought of something else: was it possible that
Sebastian's mattress might still be available for testing, and – an
even longer shot – were there still any body samples taken from
Sebastian? Even if there were, would Anne and Mike agree to
release them for analysis?

Anne Diamond hadn't come out strongly one way or another
about the Richardson hypothesis in her programmes. 'Back to
Sleep' had been her focus for the reduction of cot death, and it
had certainly helped reduce the rate in Britain. She wasn't
convinced by Richardson, but Roger Cook hoped she would be
interested in helping with his programme. She was, and what's
more, Sebastian's mattress had been kept. It was tested
immediately and antimony and phosphorus were found in
quantity. Confronted with this result, Anne and her husband gave
permission for a body sample taken from Sebastian to be analysed
as well. Roger phoned them with the result, and it was shattering:
Sebastian's body sample also contained a very high level of
antimony – in fact, the third highest of all the body samples tested
for the *Cook Report*.

The programme was due to be broadcast that night and the
'promos' had been previewing it for several days. Shocked by
the results she had received, Anne Diamond was vehement on
her BBC *Good Morning* slot:

> I was going to come on this programme and preach caution,
> caution, caution and say what the doctors want me to say –
> that there is no proven link between the antimony Roger

Cook found on mattresses and the antimony he found in some dead babies.

Today he dropped a bombshell on me. Mike and I let Roger Cook test the cot mattress Sebastian died on – and yesterday he told me they had found very high levels of antimony.

We also allowed him access to some of Sebastian's body tissue and just this morning, just a few minutes ago, Roger told me that they had found incredibly high levels of antimony in our baby.

Now I want to know why it was there. Roger has shown enough for a major, major enquiry. The Government has got to instigate a major scientific enquiry into this – and now.

'The Cot Death Poisonings', which screened at prime time throughout central England, had a sensational impact. Detailing the Richardson hypothesis, the programme gave the results of the analyses of mattresses and body samples which the *Cook Report* had commissioned. Two analysts had been involved and both were interviewed. A spokesperson for FSID appeared and was clearly disarmed by the analytical results. The programme left viewers in no doubt that the Richardson hypothesis had to be taken very seriously indeed.

During the programme Anne Diamond slammed the Department of Health. She told viewers:

> I certainly feel very angry against the Department of Health at the moment. I feel that as a parent I've been hoodwinked into believing that they thoroughly investigated the mattress theory and then dismissed it with integrity. They clearly didn't.

Viewers patently agreed with her. The *Cook Report* had foreseen that the public reaction would be overwhelming and had made arrangements for unlimited toll-free phone lines to be available from any part of Britain immediately after the programme had finished. Several teams of volunteers would be waiting to answer and the programme invited anyone with a query to phone in for advice.

And they did. Over 60,000 calls were received within 24 hours – from parents, prospective parents and bereaved parents. Many asked questions, and some told of their loss of a baby. But most of all they wanted to know: what can I do – *tonight* – to make sure my baby is safe? We told them: wrap the baby's mattress in polythene.

I was in the Birmingham studio and witnessed the scene. After Joan Shenton had telephoned me in Auckland to request an interview for the programme, I had contacted Peter Salkeld and offered to travel to Britain to assist in any way possible. He had asked me to catch the next plane.

I appeared briefly on the programme, but had been heavily involved behind the scenes providing technical back-up and liaising with Barry and the two analysts. It had been a fascinating experience. But now, manning one of the freephones after the programme, I realised what an impact the hypothesis had on parents. For so long they had been fed the idea that cot death was a medical mystery – and now, tonight, they could do something constructive themselves.

The *Cook Report* wasn't slow to realise the impact either. It was clearly onto a winner. As editor Mike Townson put it, this was the best-running story they'd ever had.

The rest of the news media nationwide in Britain pounced on it, and it dominated the news. Under headlines such as 'We're putting our babies to bed tonight on mattresses . . . and we don't know whether they will be safe or not', the press splashed the Richardson hypothesis across its pages in the days after the programme was screened. The *Daily Express* reminded its readers that as far back as 1990 it had expressed concern about chemicals used in mattresses but the Department of Health had ruled out any danger. It was reported that the Government could face legal action from parents of cot death babies over its failure to investigate the hypothesis fully in the past, and that claims against mattress manufacturers were also a possibility.

The response of the cot death establishment was varied. Individual medical researchers were highly critical of the programme, but the established cot death organisations took a more measured approach. The Scottish Cot Death Trust, while of the opinion that the *Cook Report* was not the proper forum for presenting these findings on cot death, was critical of the Government's inaction. Not prepared to sit back and wait for more research, it promptly advised parents to wrap mattresses. FSID took a similar line. They put out well considered instructions on mattress-wrapping and urged parents buying new mattresses to avoid any which contained toxic chemicals. They were concerned about the level of anxiety caused to parents by the programme, but nevertheless considered that the hypothesis was of undeniable interest and warranted further investigation.

A stronger line was taken by Dr (now Sir) Kenneth Calman, the Government's Chief Medical Officer. Describing the programme as 'limited, inadequate and flawed', he said that cot mattresses were only one of many sources of antimony in a baby's environment, and warned parents that mattress-wrapping could be dangerous. Defending the findings of the Turner Committee, he said the *Cook Report* programme had put forward nothing to invalidate them. Nevertheless, he believed that the programme had raised 'some questions which need proper investigation' and said that the Government would convene an expert group to examine the significance of trace elements.

One group, however, acted immediately: the cot mattress industry.

Responding to advance promotion of the programme, even before it went to air the largest retailer of cot mattresses in Britain, Boots, announced that they were withdrawing all their cot mattresses from sale. Bavistock withdrew 35,000 cot mattresses containing antimony, while Littlewoods and their Home Shopping division announced a temporary ban on cot mattress sales pending their review of the programme. Following the programme, John Lewis, House of Fraser, Adams Children Wear and Toys R Us all announced a suspension of sales.

Some mattress manufacturers had already removed antimony from their products following Richardson's 1989 advice, and now others rushed to do likewise. Rochingham announced that they had stopped production of mattresses containing antimony and would use a different chemical in future. There was a run on mattresses known to be free from antimony and Mothercare, who had already removed antimony in 1991, quickly sold out.

The Royal College of Midwives supported the withdrawal of cot mattresses from sale until the Department of Health could give conclusive evidence that they were safe.

'The Cot Death Poisonings' had focused only on the element antimony. This was regrettable, but understandable. The producers had selected antimony because, of the three elements phosphorus, arsenic and antimony, only antimony can be tracked meaningfully in body tissue samples. The presence of the three elements can be reliably determined in both mattresses and body samples, but in the latter an additional factor comes into play: since phosphorus and arsenic are always naturally present in body tissue, any small increase in these elements brought about from the inhalation of phosphine or arsine would not show up against the significant levels of phosphorus and arsenic which are there anyway.

Therefore, in order to demonstrate definitively that one of the three poisonous elements was in a baby's body, antimony had to be the choice. If a significant quantity of antimony *was* found in the baby's body, it could only have come from stibine gas. And the only possible source of the stibine was the baby's mattress, because – outside the chemical laboratory – stibine in significant quantity doesn't arise. In the household environment the only conceivable source is from microbiological activity on some antimonial compound, and the only source of antimonial compound in sufficient quantity would be that added to mattresses and upholstery as a fire retardant. If, therefore, antimony was found to be present in the baby's mattress as well as its body, the conclusion that the baby had died of stibine poisoning would be almost inescapable.

In the event, the focus on antimony in 'The Cot Death Poisonings' had a disadvantage because it drew attention away from the fact that cot death could be caused not only by stibine but also by phosphine and arsine. And there was no doubt that phosphorus and arsenic could equally well be present in a baby's mattress. Indeed, in certain countries (for example, New Zealand and Australia) phosphorus and arsenic were more likely to be present in a baby's cot than antimony.

Even more confusing for the lay person was the fact that commentators responding to the *Cook Report* drew attention to the relatively low toxicity of antimony. But it wasn't antimony which poisoned the babies – it was *stibine*, the intensely toxic gas *derived* from antimony. This technical distinction seemed to escape virtually all the critics of the *Cook Report*.

Nevertheless, for the moment the spotlight was on antimony. No-one questioned that it was present in many cot mattresses – that was common knowledge. And no-one could question that antimony had been found in the bodies of cot death babies. But critics of the programme were quick to ask: Had the body antimony killed the baby? And even if it had, how could you tell that it came from the mattress? Wasn't antimony in all sorts of things around the house?

10

Follow-up

Once an in-depth television programme goes to air and the tension is over, the studio can become a rather festive place. On this occasion it was apparently more festive than usual. The *Cook Report* regarded 'The Cot Death Poisonings' as probably their best programme to date, and they'd been making programmes for years.

Barry was also in the studio when the programme was screened. We were enjoying the champagne and hors-d'oeuvres along with everyone else, but we had something else on our minds: a follow-up programme.

Even at the production stage it was obvious that 'The Cot Death Poisonings' was going to be a success. The research behind the programme had broken totally new ground. Nobody – anywhere, it seemed – had analysed tissue samples from cot death babies for antimony. Consequently, nobody had made the link between tissue samples and the babies' own mattresses. It was scarcely credible that even in Britain, where over the preceding 40 years some 60,000 babies had died of cot death, almost all subject to autopsy and an inquest, no-one (except Barry Richardson) had thought to test body samples for *any* poison.

Not only was the analytical programme new, but the results made compelling viewing. The producers were ecstatic. But television being what it is, they thought the subject was finished so far as they were concerned. They were already thinking about next week's programme.

Barry and I had other ideas. We wanted a follow-up programme to reinforce the hypothesis in viewers' minds, and that night we put this to Peter Salkeld. 'Fine,' he said, 'but we're not going over that ground again. You've got to think of something new.'

It didn't take us long. 'The Cot Death Poisonings' had proved the presence of unexpectedly high levels of antimony in the bodies of many cot death babies. If antimony in mattresses had resulted in antimony in dead babies, then – if the hypothesis was correct – there must also be living babies and toddlers with antimony in their bodies. The only difference was that the living babies had not received a lethal dose of stibine. If we could find significant amounts of antimony in the bodies of living infants, it would be powerful evidence supporting the hypothesis.

The question was: how to collect body samples for analysis from living infants? At first Barry suggested analysing fingernails, but babies don't have much in the way of fingernails. We hit on analysing their hair.

Whenever human beings ingest toxic elements, the body tries to excrete them. In some cases, it can't excrete them efficiently – for example, lead, cadmium and mercury accumulate in the body, mostly in the skeleton; but others, like copper and manganese, are readily excreted. For centuries it has been known that arsenic is excreted mainly into the hair and fingernails; and arsenic, of course, was a popular poison in earlier times. It was analysis of a single hair taken from the body of Napoleon Bonaparte which proved that he had been poisoned with arsenic.

Antimony, the next member of Group Vb to arsenic, behaves in the same way. The body excretes it mainly into the hair and fingernails.

We explained to Peter Salkeld our idea of taking hair samples from babies and analysing them for antimony. This would be a new angle, not to mention a worthwhile piece of research which had not been carried out before. The *Cook Report* agreed to run with it and provide research back-up and filming facilities. But there were no promises of a programme. They would wait and see what we came up with, and there was a potential slot in two weeks' time. It would be a tight schedule.

The best place to round up a sufficient number of babies and toddlers was in housing estates, where the population density is high and young families congregate. The persuasive Joan Shenton pulled some rank and quickly organised for mothers and children to be at four community centres in different parts of the country. District nurses would take the samples. We wanted as many samples of hair from infants and toddlers as possible. But it would also be important to collect hair samples from babies' mothers: since the mothers hadn't been sleeping on the cot mattresses, their hair would contain only 'ambient' antimony and would therefore act as 'control' samples.

Criticism was voiced and in two towns official pressure forced the district nurse and the community centre to pull out, but sampling in Derby and Oxford went ahead.

Over 70 samples of babies' hair were collected, together with approximately 20 hair samples taken from mothers, and these were sent to Ron Rooney, the analyst who had tested cot mattresses for 'The Cot Death Poisonings'.

Programme deadline was approaching, and when we still hadn't received the test results, I phoned Ron. He had done the analyses but didn't want to send the results until the next day. Having been an analytical chemist for over 50 years, I knew what that meant: he wanted to run the tests again, just to be sure.

The test results were sensational. Levels of antimony in hair from many of the babies and toddlers were 10–50 times higher than the typical levels in the mothers' hair. In one case, the concentration in a child's hair was over 100 times that in its mother's hair.

The result was inescapable: babies and toddlers were clearly being exposed to antimony at levels which other members of their household were not experiencing. And not just a little bit more antimony – the average level in the children's hair was 26 times greater than the average level for mothers.

Dr Calman had tried to explain away the presence of significant amounts of antimony in babies' bodies, saying that antimony was common – present in food, water and tobacco smoke – and implying that a bit of antimony in a mattress would make no difference. In truth, antimony is very rare in the domestic environment, the only significant source being mattresses, upholstery materials, etc. Obviously these *did* make a difference: they were the only conceivable explanation for the huge discrepancy in the antimony levels between the living babies and their mothers.

But not all the living babies had high amounts of antimony in their hair. Some had virtually none. So the argument applied in reverse: if some babies' hair contained minuscule amounts of antimony, and all babies were exposed to only ambient antimony, why didn't *all* the babies' hair show a minuscule amount of antimony – or, for that matter, all show a high amount? Whatever the result in babies' hair – whether low- or high-level antimony – exposure to 'ambient' antimony must result in similar levels across all babies.

It was evident that some babies were getting antimony into their bodies from a 'non-ambient' source. And antimony in any quantity is available to the body only via stibine gas. A baby can't just suck antimony into its body from its mattress – the antimonial compounds don't work that way. They have to be converted to gas first, and the only way that can happen is by the action of a suitable fungus. This action of fungus on antimonial compounds won't occur under normal household conditions. It will only occur where conditions are favourable: warm, humid and moist – just like a baby's cot.

The hair analyses were another confirmation of the Richardson hypothesis, and the *Cook Report* team were impressed. They decided to screen a second programme and 'The Cot Death Poisonings – Part 2' went to air on 1 December 1994.

This programme dealt briefly again with the hypothesis, but concentrated on the hair analyses. Once more the *Cook Report* threw its weight behind Richardson's findings. And this time, the programme included a hands-on demonstration of how to wrap a mattress to block out any poisonous gas.

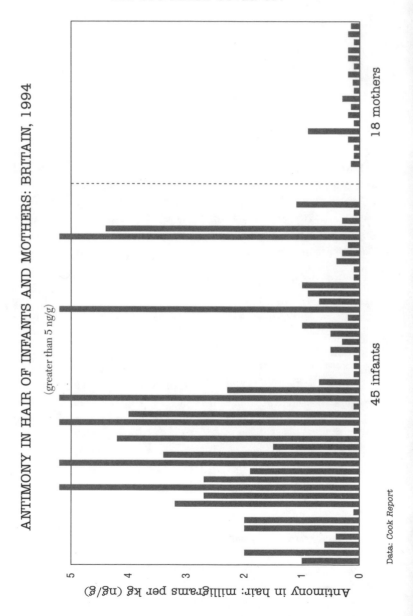

ANTIMONY IN HAIR OF INFANTS AND MOTHERS: BRITAIN, 1994

(greater than 5 ng/g)

Antimony in hair: milligrams per kg (ng/g)

45 infants

18 mothers

Data: *Cook Report*

ANTIMONY IN HAIR OF INFANTS AND MOTHERS: BRITAIN, 1994

After the *Cook Report* analyses in 1994 had shown high levels of antimony in the liver samples of a number of cot death babies, it was realised that many living babies and toddlers might also have antimony in their bodies, arising from sublethal doses of stibine from their mattresses.

Antimony arising from chronic but sublethal exposure is excreted by the body into the hair. Hair samples were taken from 45 infants up to two years of age and analysed for antimony. To provide a control, hair samples were taken from the mothers of 18 of these infants and analysed.

The results can only be described as staggering.

First, they refute Dr Calman's assertion that antimony is widespread in the environment. If this were so, the mothers and babies would show similar levels of antimony in their hair.

Secondly, the hair of 10 of the infants did not contain any detectable antimony, and a further 6 contained a relatively low level, more or less comparable with the adults' hair. These infants and the mothers had been exposed to 'background' antimony.

However, the remaining 29 infants had much higher levels of antimony in their hair than the mothers; in fact, 5 of them had more than 5ng/g (some as much as 50ng/g), and 1 had 100ng/g.

The confirmation of the Richardson hypothesis is apparent from these results: some infants are exposed to antimony from a source in their environment to which their mothers are not exposed; this source can only be the mattress on which they sleep; and the only means of transfer of the antimony into their bodies is as stibine.

The long term effect of excessive antimony in the bodies of infants is not known.

Interviewed on the programme about his analytical results for hair, Ron Rooney said:

> I was surprised at how high the [antimony levels in] babies were, related to their mothers. Mother has had much more time to accumulate antimony (admittedly it grows out with hair), but the average baby was 20 times as high as its mother. It ranged up to a hundred times. The average over the range of babies was 3800 parts per billion [of antimony]; the average mother was 165 [parts per billion].

As for Dr Calman's assertion that babies could get antimony from all sorts of places, Ron Rooney disposed of this in short order. Knowing that Calman was wrong, he had analysed a range of fresh and processed baby food, baby shampoo, cigarettes and a sample of the local water supply. Antimony was not detectable in the water, the shampoo, or any of the food except for minute quantities in some canned baby dinners containing meat. As for the cigarettes, no antimony could be detected in new cigarette tobacco, but there was a small amount of antimony in filters of cigarettes which had been smoked. It appeared, however, that this antimony may have been a constituent of the filter material itself, rather than absorbed from the smoke into the filter; in such a circumstance a baby would not be exposed to any antimony. (This is not to say that all cigarette tobacco is free from antimony; the possibility of antimony being present in some cigarette smoke cannot be excluded.)

Ron Rooney's results were exactly what he expected. As he later expressed it, antimony comprises just one part per million (0.0001%) of the earth – hardly everywhere around us!

Professor Thomas West, who had served on the Turner Committee, commented on the results of the hair analyses:

> The conclusion is obviously that the baby is exposed to a hazard or a risk that the mother is not exposed to; or that babies are particularly susceptible to antimony or arsenic or whatever it is that's causing the problem. And if that's the

case, then there's only one solution to the problem, and that is to take these fire retardants right out of the environment in which the baby sleeps.

There was an extra twist to this programme. Now that high levels of antimony had been confirmed in living babies, parents had something else to be concerned about: exposure to stibine might not have caused a child to die of cot death, but what would be the effects as the child grew up? Professor Derek Bryce-Smith, Emeritus Professor of Chemistry, had broached this matter in the programme:

> There might be no obvious symptoms, but if we're getting toxic substances transferred to the brain in non-lethal amounts, these could cause – in principle – impairment of learning ability, impairment of behavioural control . . . So there's the potential for nasty things to happen.

In the publicity which followed the second programme the questions became: My child didn't die of cot death but it did sleep on a cot mattress. Could it have antimony in its body, and if so, what will the effect of that be? These questions went unanswered. (I certainly had my suspicions, based upon the known effects of long- term exposure to antimony, but was asked by the *Cook Report* not to spell these out publicly. The programme had caused quite enough mayhem as it was.)

But there were other unanswered questions, of a quite different nature, which were finally solved as a direct result of the *Cook Report* analyses. Between the two programmes, as thousands of people contacted the studio, a particular group of parents came to light: those who had been put under suspicion of mistreating their babies in some way.

When parents lose a baby through unexplained death, the police are informed and they interview the parents. It's not a task the police relish, but in Britain it has led to cot death parents being accused of murdering their babies. While it is rare for prosecutions to result, the very accusation leaves a scar. The suspicion lingers and the social stigma is pervasive. Losing a baby for no apparent cause is bad enough, but to be accused of murdering it is horrific – and at one time it was being suggested that 10% of all unexplained infant deaths were actually murders.

The *Cook Report* investigations explained how these injustices could come about. There is little doubt that many parents who have lost a child to cot death have been wrongfully accused of smothering it, whereas in fact the child was poisoned.

Other instances came to light as well: parents whose babies had not died but had been unwell and had red blotches on their skin. Mothers would take them to the doctor; and the doctor, suspicious of abuse, would report the matter to the police. In some cases babies had as a result been forcibly removed from their families and placed in foster care. In others, the mother had been denied access to the baby except under supervision. It was pretty rough stuff.

Out of the *Cook Report* tests came the answer. The visible signs of 'abuse' on the baby reported by the doctor were not bruises at all: they were red marks on the skin, known as 'petechiae', a frequent result of stibine poisoning. The baby had been a 'near miss'. (Petechiae are common where babies have died of cot death. Pathologists have frequently reported them.)

Not all of these incidents could be followed up by the *Cook Report* team – after all, that is not the task of a television studio. Nevertheless two were investigated.

One of these involved a mother whose baby daughter had been taken into foster care. The baby had survived a series of 'near misses', and the doctor, baffled by the repeated breathing problems, called in an expert. After analysing recordings of breathing monitors and secretly videoing the mother, the expert concluded that she had been attempting to suffocate the baby. By the time the *Cook Report* learned of this, the baby was back with her family. Eventually – after the diagnoses of five other doctors and a Court battle – the baby had been restored to her parents, but only on condition that a lock was put on her bedroom door and that she was never left alone with her mother.

The mother still had the baby's original cot mattress and she submitted it for testing. The *Cook Report* team was not surprised to find that the PVC mattress cover contained a very high level of antimony, almost certainly accounting for the series of 'near misses'. Furthermore, hair analysis showed that the child had five times as much antimony in her hair as her mother did. There was no doubt that the child had experienced chronic exposure to antimony in her home environment, but never a fatal dose.

While not investigated by the *Cook Report*, another case – still not resolved – came to my personal attention. A Birmingham family had two children and then lost the third to cot death. There was a strong suspicion of murder, and although there was no prosecution, the matter hit the headlines of the local newspaper. The father, a chef with sixteen years' work record with the one employer, lost his job and spent the next two years on the dole, unable to find any employment.

There had been an autopsy and post-mortem samples taken. The mattress had been disposed of but the post-mortem samples were still being held at a local hospital. I decided to follow it up personally.

The pathologist's report stated that in his opinion the death was not due to natural causes but was the result of suffocation. He gave evidence at the inquest and the coroner duly issued a report which read: 'Cause of death: Suffocation by overlaying. Verdict: Misadventure.' The family hotly denied the allegation of overlaying.

But tucked away in the pathologist's report is a pivotal observation: that he found on the baby 'scattered subepicardial petechiae', in other words, red blotches under the skin – the same red blotches which, when found in other babies, had led to allegations of physical abuse but had actually been caused by exposure to stibine.

The next step was obvious: to have the post-mortem samples analysed for antimony. The parents gave their wholehearted approval, so I approached the Birmingham Coroner, asking for the samples to be released to an independent analyst. My repeated requests met with repeated refusals. The coroner gave as his reason: 'In the present case, given the verdict which was recorded, I believe it would be inappropriate to accede to your request.'

It is clear from the pathologist's report that no chemical analysis of post-mortem samples was carried out. If such analysis might clear the parents' name and give a lead as to the cause of death, one wonders why the samples weren't released. After all, the coroner has a duty to determine the cause of death if at all possible.

Or does the Birmingham Coroner want to avoid the possibility of antimony being found? Would such a finding cause embarrassment to the coroner and the pathologist?

This sort of legal roundabout can go on for years.

The immediate outcome of the *Cook Report* analyses was that by the time the second programme was over, the link between antimony and cot death had been established:

> Antimony was present in many cot mattresses
> It was found in many cot death babies – a lot of it
> It was also found in many living babies – a lot of it
> But it wasn't found in their mothers to any great extent.

In Barry Richardson's experience, the livers of non-cot death babies usually contained less than 2 nanograms of antimony per gram of liver, and never exceeded 10ng/g; but some cot death babies had shown levels in excess of 100ng/g, and even higher levels in lung tissue, up to 1000ng/g. Antimony undeniably had a link with cot death, and the only source at these levels was the baby's cot.

But antimony wasn't the whole story. Phosphorus and arsenic had been overlooked in the furore – and both of these were more dangerous than antimony. And far more widespread, especially in New Zealand and Australia.

11

The British Government Acts

The immediate reaction of the British Chief Medical Officer, Dr Kenneth Calman, to the first *Cook Report* was to try and tough it out. Stating that the programme didn't stand up to scientific examination, he said there were no plans to change existing Government guidelines on cot mattresses.

He even went so far as to say that the programme's recommendation to wrap mattresses would put at risk more babies' lives than would be at risk from antimony. (He would soon change his tune. Two weeks later, in company with FSID, he was telling parents that if they were worried, they should wrap their mattresses.)

For her part, Health Secretary Virginia Bottomley remarked that television producers making scientific programmes which could arouse public alarm should first obtain expert advice from the Department of Health. Junior Health Minister, Tom Sackville, attacked the *Cook Report* for being 'highly irresponsible' and frightening thousands of mothers. Repeating Dr Calman's line that antimony was widespread, he called the programme 'sensationalism, made by a journalist with no scientific or medical expertise whatsoever' – as if Roger Cook had made the programme on his own!

Despite his knee-jerk reaction of rubbishing the first *Cook Report* programme, Dr Calman knew he had a problem. The media frenzy and level of public concern were such that he had to take some action. Having signalled on 19 November that he would convene an expert group to examine the significance of antimony, he announced on 30 November that such a group had been set up to steer further work on cot death within the Department of Health.

The task of the Expert Group to Investigate Cot Death Theories would be to review the findings of the Turner Committee and investigate information which had come to light since May 1991 linking antimony with cot death.

When Dr Calman announced the composition of the Group (known as the Limerick Committee), it certainly looked eminently qualified to carry out its task. The Countess of Limerick CBE, Chairman of the British Red Cross, was to chair it. Among its members were three paediatricians, two Professors of Chemistry and a Professor of Public Health Medicine, a microbiologist, a poisons expert, a cot death researcher, a midwife and a magistrate. On the face of it, a highly suitable line-up. Dr Calman publicly expressed his gratitude that these people were prepared to embark on the task.

But the membership rang instant alarm bells among those who believed the Richardson hypothesis. Even making allowance for the fact that in such a specialised area of research the field of available experts for the Department to call upon was necessarily limited, this particular grouping seemed less than desirable.

Lady Limerick wasn't just involved in the Red Cross; she was also Vice-Chairman of FSID. The cot death researcher, Dr Shireen Chantler, was an employee of FSID and also secretary of its Scientific Advisory Committee. And FSID had been denouncing the Richardson hypothesis for years now.

One of the Committee's paediatricians, Dr Jean Keeling, was on the grant review panel of FSID. Together with the poisons expert, Dr Alex Proudfoot, she had been a member of the Turner Committee.

Of particular concern was the very influential secretariat which would assist the Committee. There was little doubt that this would include Mr P. G. Dibb, who had been Administrative Secretary for the Turner Committee and had assiduously supported that Committee's findings. He turned up as

Administrative Secretary for the Limerick Committee as well.

It was my view that anyone connected with, for example, FSID or the Turner Committee, should decline appointment to the new Committee.

Furthermore, the Committee appeared to have technical limitations, as Barry Richardson pointed out in the second *Cook Report* programme:

> This is an environmental and toxicological problem and unfortunately the new group doesn't have the necessary expertise. The information that has been issued recently by the Government indicates that they don't understand the problem at all.

All up, the Richardson camp were appalled at the personnel chosen for the Committee. And – as events would show – with good reason.

It wasn't long before some members of the Committee were making public statements which appeared to me to be inappropriate, given the fact that the Committee had been set up to investigate the very issue upon which these members were commenting.

FSID's measured response to the first *Cook Report* programme evaporated. On 2 December they slated the second programme in a press release:

> The second *Cook Report* added nothing to the sum of knowledge about cot death. It has served only to confuse and terrorize the public even more . . .

Dr Shireen Chantler was quoted:

> The Foundation has commissioned, and has invited applications for, research in this area since 1990 including invitations issued to Barry Richardson . . . Send us sound scientific proposals – proposals that will answer the kind of unanswered questions displayed across the television screens of the nation for the past two weeks – and we will do the job.

On 5 December Lady Limerick was a guest on a BBC Radio 4 programme, where she said that the Richardson hypothesis was unproven because it had not been shown by the *Cook Report* that the antimony had come from the cot mattresses; antimony could arise from the normal environment.

Professor Peter Fleming, one of the paediatricians on the Committee and regarded as the doyen of the cot death establishment in Britain, was hot off the mark, in the company of Professor Michael Cooke (also a Committee member) and Dr Chantler. Responding directly to the *Cook Report* programmes, they published in the *British Medical Journal* of 17 December an article denying central aspects of the hypothesis.

Professor Fleming was in print again – in *The Lancet* this time – on 18 March 1995, categorically denying the hypothesis. Then he hit the television airwaves, in a BBC *QED* programme on 21 March, quoting from interim results obtained from the CESDI (Confidential Enquiry into Stillbirths and Deaths in Infancy) study.[*]

Professor Michael Cooke had his turn. By 6 December he had publicly described the *Cook Report* programmes as 'blatant scaremongering'.

Professor Gordon Fell also got into the act. As well as being a member of the Committee, he acted as a consultant to the Scottish Cot Death Trust. The Trust had carried out tests to measure antimony levels in samples of liver tissue, and on the basis of the results went public in March 1995 with a categorical denial of the Richardson hypothesis – a denial which, as their press release made clear, was totally supported by Professor Fell.

By April 1995 I had had enough. I wrote a formal letter to the Secretary of State for Health, reminding her that the Limerick

---

[*] The CESDI project, a major case/control epidemiological study, was established by the British Government in January 1993. It has studied every infant death in the Avon, Trent and Yorkshire health authority areas since its inception. Parents are asked over 500 questions. The study is still ongoing.

Committee were supposed to be carrying out an impartial investigation into the Richardson hypothesis and that all these public statements were, in my opinion, evidence of pre-determination of the issue. If they didn't modify their behaviour, they would be likely to face judicial review of their findings. (Judicial review is a Court procedure where a Judge decides whether a public body has carried out its functions properly. In the case of the Limerick Committee, one possible outcome of judicial review would be the setting aside of its final report.) I quoted a passage from *Halsbury's Laws of England* which appeared to me to be relevant:

> Likelihood of bias may . . . arise because an adjudicator . . . has made known his views about the merits of the very issue or issues of a similar nature in such a way as to suggest prejudgment, or because he is so actively associated with the . . . conduct of proceedings before him, either in his personal capacity or by virtue of his membership of an interested organisation, as to make himself in substance, both judge and party . . . It is generally unnecessary to establish the presence of actual bias.

The letter seemed to have an effect. It appeared that the Committee became more circumspect and that individual members tempered their public pronouncements. Lady Limerick may not have liked it, but she clearly reined them in.

In July 1995 I visited Lady Limerick at the Red Cross head office in London. Lady Limerick is a gracious person, not outwardly conscious of her position in the aristocracy, and she was keen to hear what I had to say. It was a worthwhile meeting, albeit stormy at times. As would be expected, we discussed the hypothesis at length. She asked many perceptive questions and it was clear that she had a good grasp of chemistry.

My aim in meeting Lady Limerick wasn't to stop the Committee in their tracks. Obviously, they had to work through their testing regime; this was part of their terms of reference. But there was something the Committee could do in the meantime, which would be of immense importance. Bearing in mind the success in reducing the cot death rate which had followed Richardson's advice, and the undeniable results of the *Cook Report* testing for antimony in mattresses and body samples, would the Committee publicly endorse mattress-wrapping, just as a precaution?

Mattress-wrapping was cheap, easy and demonstrably safe. If the hypothesis turned out to be wrong, no harm would have been done by wrapping mattresses. But if the hypothesis was right, failure to wrap mattresses would result in needless cot deaths.

I put the question to Lady Limerick: could she state categorically that the hypothesis was wrong? If she couldn't, then a refusal to endorse mattress-wrapping was tantamount to gambling with babies' lives.

Even though she agreed that the Richardson hypothesis might be correct, she refused my request point blank. And her reason? That the Committee would lose credibility with the scientific community. I asked what the scientific community had to do with it – what about the babies? But this argument fell upon deaf ears.

As I wrote to Lady Limerick in July 1994 after our meeting:

> Your Group was set up, very precipitately, as the Government's answer to the *Cook Report* programmes, with the purpose of answering the very proper questions and concerns of the public. It is funded with public money, not research grants from some scientific or private establishment. There was no mention in the terms of reference of convincing the scientific community.
>
> I suggest that your responsibility is to the public at large, not some unnamed academics. This is not a study of some arcane philosophical question. The lives and deaths of many babies are the stakes.

During our meeting I had made the offer to Lady Limerick to assist the Committee on technical matters and explain the chemistry and toxicology involved. But we had reached a stand-off, which continues to the present. In the meantime, the Committee have carried out laboratory trials in an attempt to replicate Richardson's work. These trials have been technically flawed, as I point out in Chapter 12 of this book, which deals with the chemistry of the hypothesis in detail.

If the Committee reject the Richardson hypothesis in their final report, they will certainly have some difficulty answering the following questions:

- Why wasn't cot death identified as a specific phenomenon until 1953, following the introduction of cot mattress covers containing antimony and phosphorus?

- Why did the cot death rate increase in parallel with the increasing use of antimony and phosphorus in mattresses?

- Why has face-up sleeping reduced the cot death rate?

- Why did the cot death rate in Britain dive before 'Back to Sleep' was adopted there?

- Wasn't this due to the publicising of the Richardson hypothesis?

The outcome of the Limerick Committee's investigations could have far-reaching ramifications. It came as no surprise that immediately following the screening of the *Cook Report* programmes a number of lawyers sprang into action. On 1 December 1994 it was announced that the Law Society and the Legal Aid Board had taken steps to prepare for mass legal claims by parents of cot death babies. Parents were invited to get in touch with a team of solicitors who would co-ordinate the claims, and by 9 December over 40 sets of parents had done so.

According to one lawyer, cot death parents appeared to have a strong case against mattress manufacturers under the Consumer Protection Act 1987. In his words:

You don't have to prove that [the mattress was] the sole cause of the baby's death; you don't have to prove that the manufacturer could have foreseen the problem; and you don't have to prove that they lacked care.

Damages could be up to £7,500 for bereavement, with the possibility of other damages being awarded as well, and there was no need to wait for medical or scientific consensus on the cause of cot death before filing a claim.

In addition, it was envisaged that mattress manufacturers could be prosecuted under the new General Product Safety Regulations, which had come into force on 3 October 1994. These Regulations made it an offence to place on the market a product which was not safe, especially when that product was used by children.

Of greater significance for the Government is the potential for claims by bereaved parents against the Department of Health, on two counts: first, for failing to investigate the Richardson hypothesis fully when they first became aware of it; and secondly, for failing to advise parents to cover cot mattresses with polythene. After all, the Secretary of State for Health in the early 1990s, Virginia Bottomley, flatly denied that there was any merit in the Richardson hypothesis at all.

If the Limerick Committee are forced in the end to admit that the Richardson hypothesis is correct, such claims against the Government will become a distinct possibility.

In my view, the concept of yet another Department of Health Expert Group to investigate the Richardson hypothesis was flawed from the outset. By late 1994 the matter was completely polarised. Anyone who was anybody in the cot death field had a view on Richardson's work – often a fixed view. Rather than a departmental Expert Group, there should have been a Commission of Inquiry before an experienced judicial officer. The Limerick Committee could have done all the research they wanted, just as Barry Richardson had done. And then – just like

Barry, and FSID, and anyone else – they could have presented it as witnesses before the Commission and been subject to cross-examination.

At the time of writing (June 1996), the Limerick Committee are nineteen months into their investigations. They commissioned a testing programme and in December 1995 issued their first interim report, based on the results. According to this report, Barry Richardson's experiments could not be replicated and, furthermore, Barry had misinterpreted his own original findings. In the words of the Limerick Committee: 'At all stages of our deliberations we have asked the question "is there any evidence of risk to infants?" To date we have seen none.'

A careful reading of the interim report reveals that they've got a long way to go:

- They are awaiting information from the expanded CESDI study on the chemicals and micro-organisms present in cot mattresses. These results will not be available until late 1996.

- They have not determined whether there is a link between cot death and fire-retardant chemicals – again, information due in late 1996.

- They have not finished their investigation of the relevance and source of excessive antimony found in the hair of living infants and in the post-mortem body tissue of cot death babies.

Barry Richardson hit the nail on the head: 'It seems irresponsible for the Group to present conclusions on which the public will rely, and to permit publication of papers with similar conclusions, before completion of their investigations.' Quite so. The interim report did appear at the time to be premature.

It now transpires that in February 1996 the Limerick Committee were considering the possibility that Barry Richardson was right after all. They were still looking into the fungal generation of stibine from antimony fire retardants. Perhaps the Committee are revisiting the conclusion on the

Richardson hypothesis which they announced in their interim report of December 1995. If so, the interim report was definitely premature.

The Committee have other research in train and do not expect to publish their final report until early 1997.

By which time, it won't matter what the Limerick Committee report, whether they report, when they report, or even if they report. Their deliberations will have been overtaken by events in New Zealand.

12

For the Technically Minded

This account would be incomplete without a technical exposition of the Richardson hypothesis and the attempts which have been made to replicate his initial work. In this chapter I set out the chemistry of the matter. Technical terms are used but the text is not diverted with explanations of their meaning. I would encourage the lay reader not to give up on this chapter for want of a degree in chemistry; it all becomes clear in the end!

The mobilisation of arsenic into the gaseous phase was first observed in the 1820s but the identity of these gases could not at that time be elucidated. In 1874 Selmi suggested that a fungus produced nascent hydrogen, reacting with basic copper arsenate to form arsine.

In 1892 Gosio demonstrated that the gas comprised either arsenic trihydride or alkyl homologues of the trihydride, and that these gases were produced by fungal activity on the basic copper arsenate compounds. Just which alkyl homologues was not clear to him, but he considered that they were combinations of the methyl and ethyl compounds. Subsequent work, however, demonstrated that the principal compounds of this reaction are arsine (arsenic trihydride) and/or the trimethyl derivative.

The mobilisation of arsenic by fungal activity was later used as an analytical method for the detection of trace amounts of arsenic, this technique being more sensitive and more specific than the classical qualitative methods employed at the time (the early 1900s). Around the same time it was suggested that this technique could also be used as a sensitive means for detecting phosphorus and antimony.

By the time Gosio became involved, the structure of the Periodic Table had been well accepted and it was recognised that nitrogen, phosphorus, arsenic, antimony and bismuth fell into Group V/Vb.

It had long been known that organic compounds of nitrogen were converted to ammonia by microbiological action but it seems that little interest was taken in the gaseous mobilisation of the other elements of the group, except for the formation of phosphine and the dimer of phosphine (phosphorus dihydride), which arose in marsh gas. Will-o'-the-wisp, the flickering flame often observed at night over marshlands, is caused by the combustion of biologically produced methane, but the source of the ignition remained obscure until it was discovered that phosphine was also present in this methane. At the time it was thought that phosphine was spontaneously flammable and that this caused the ignition of the methane.

Phosphine was generated in the laboratory by J. B. Dumas and others last century but the pure gas did not ignite spontaneously, and it was then realised that it was phosphorus dihydride which was the igniting gas.

The significance of these discoveries about the hydrides of phosphorus is that – parallel with the gaseous arsenic compounds – they too are produced by microbiological activity on compounds of the element in question.

The fact that the elements arsenic, nitrogen and phosphorus acted in a similar fashion came as no surprise. The electron structures of the two outer orbits of the three elements are the same and it had long been known that, as elements of the same group and therefore the same valencies, they exhibit many similar properties.

Little attention appears to have been paid to the gaseous mobilisation of antimony by microbiological activity, presumably because of the rarity of this element in the earth's crust. Stibine had been generated chemically in the laboratory during the nineteenth century and its chemistry was quite well known. It had been observed that, like phosphorus, antimony formed a dihydride; and further that these hydrides of antimony, like those of phosphorus, were very unstable compounds.

The first specific reference to the mobilisation of antimony by microbiological activity appears to arise from research by Challenger and Barnard in the 1940s. They added phenylstibonic acid as the sodium salt to cultures of moulds on breadcrumbs and allowed them to incubate in air. The volatile products were found to contain antimony.

As with the generation of hydrides of phosphorus above marshland, methylated derivatives of antimony are detected above the mud of estuaries. Large quantities of similar compounds of other metals are produced in estuarine mud by microbiological activity (for example, lead tetraethyl).

After the lengthy investigations by Challenger and Barnard, it seems that no further research was carried out into the mobilisation of antimony by microbiological activity until Richardson became involved in 1989. Although his work has since been questioned and is the subject of continuing study, he conclusively demonstrated the generation of stibine and/or its alkyl homologues by fungal action on compounds of antimony in cot mattresses on which babies had died of cot death. Others have also done so, but only intermittently.

As would be expected, the fifth member of the Group V/Vb elements, bismuth, also forms a trihydride, but there does not appear to be any research to suggest that this compound can be formed by fungal activity.

The crux of the Richardson hypothesis is that there is one prime cause of cot death: poisoning by one or more of the gases phosphine, arsine and stibine and/or their lower alkyl homologues, the gases being produced by fungal activity on compounds of the elements phosphorus, arsenic and antimony respectively which are present either naturally or by deliberate addition in the mattress on which the baby sleeps. These gases all exhibit anticholinesterase activity, and as such interfere with the destruction of acetylcholine at the synapses of the nervous system. The accumulation of acetylcholine inhibits the passage of nerve impulses from the brain to the heart and lungs, resulting in slowing and eventual cessation of heart function and of breathing.

The sources of the elements occurring in a baby's environment include compounds in mattresses (both cot mattresses and adult mattresses) which contain:

phosphorus: naturally present in many natural fibres, ti-tree bark, coconut fibre, sheepskins and fleece wool

added as a fabric conditioning agent, fire retardant, plasticiser and catalyst

residues from synthetic detergents

arsenic: naturally present in some sheepskins and fleece wool, some natural fibres and some tree bark

added as a biocide

present as an impurity in antimony

antimony: naturally present in some sheepskins and fleece wool, and some tree bark

added as a fire retardant and as a catalyst

Several fungi have the capacity to convert compounds of these elements into the respective gases described above, but by far the most important is *Scopulariopsis brevicaulis*. Other organisms which have been shown to have this capacity include *Mucor mucedo* and *Penicillium notatum*.

S. brevicaulis grows readily on protein substrates and it is for this reason that the characteristic ammoniacal odour is detected above cheeses, milk and meat which have become contaminated by this fungus. Most moulds prefer carbohydrates as their food source, but it seems that *S. brevicaulis* consumes more protein than is necessary for the production of its own protein needs and disposes of the excess nitrogen from the protein as either ammonia or trimethylamine.

As observed above, there is a marked chemical similarity between nitrogen and the elements phosphorus, arsenic and antimony, and *S. brevicaulis* consumes compounds of these elements in the same manner as it does nitrogenous compounds. In the case of the latter three elements, these are not required by the fungus for its metabolism; the fungus consumes the compounds to obtain the associated carbon, hydrogen and oxygen in the food source for energy production. The phosphorus, arsenic and antimony are waste, indeed toxic, for the mould, and so must be excreted. This is achieved in exactly the same manner as for excess nitrogen, namely, conversion to a corresponding gas.

It is these gases which poison babies.

At first sight it might be thought that nitrogen, phosphorus, arsenic and antimony are widely differing elements, so far as the anticholinesterase activity of their trihydrides is concerned, since their respective atomic numbers are 7, 15, 33 and 51, and their respective atomic weights are 14, 31, 75 and 122. The atomic volumes of the elements, however, are the significant parameter, and these are not widely different. On the scale of 5 units (for beryllium, the smallest element) to 70 (for caesium, the largest) the relative atomic volumes of the four Group V/Vb elements are 14 (nitrogen), 15 (phosphorus), 16 (arsenic) and 18 (antimony). As a consequence, an organic radical containing one of the three latter elements is not very different either volumetrically or structurally from a similar compound of nitrogen. The fungal enzyme systems capable of assimilating a suitable nitrogenous compound could well be equally capable of assimilating suitable compounds of phosphorus, arsenic and antimony; hence the evolution of the toxic gases from these three elements by *S. brevicaulis*.

At this point it is worth noting that the trihydride gases of the first four elements of Group V/Vb also have widely varying vapour densities. The figures are:

Gas	Molecular weight	Vapour density	Relative to air = 1	Diffusion rate stibine = 1
ammonia	17	8.5	0.59	2.62
phosphine	34	17	1.18	1.85
arsine	78	39	2.71	1.23
stibine	125	62.5	4.34	1.00

From this it is clear why ammonia, being substantially less dense than air, is sometimes smelt in the air above a baby's cot. The other three gases, all being more dense than air, will lie on the mattress or flow down off its edges. This applies especially to arsine and stibine and accounts for the benefit of face-up sleeping.

Face-up sleeping also assists to some extent against poisoning by phosphine; but owing to the relatively small difference in density between phosphine and air, face-up sleeping is less effective than for the more dense gases. For example, the ambient temperature in a baby's cot can reach 40°C and the ambient temperature of a room in winter can be as low as 10°C; under these conditions the density of phosphine on the cot mattress, relative to air, is reduced to 1.07 and it will readily diffuse in the warm air to reach the baby's face, even if the baby is sleeping face up.

It is this difference in the respective densities of the three gases which accounts for the fact that face-up sleeping has achieved only partial success in eliminating cot death. At the outset, adoption of face-up sleeping was very effective in both New Zealand and Britain in reducing the cot death rate (although in Britain the rate had been falling steadily over the 2¹/₂-year period between the publication of the Richardson hypothesis in June 1989 and the official launch of 'Back to Sleep' in December 1991). In New Zealand face-up sleeping achieved ostensibly better results than it did in Britain, because New Zealand had been denied the prior benefit of Richardson's findings.

In both countries, however, the reduction in cot death achieved by face-up sleeping has levelled off. The reason is that while antimony has been largely eliminated as a hazard in Britain and has probably never been such a serious hazard in New Zealand, antimony was only one of the contributing elements, and face-up sleeping is not very effective against phosphine.

Breathing in a gas is not the only way in which it can reach a baby's bloodstream; it can be absorbed through the skin as well. The skin of a baby is much more permeable than that of an adult, because a baby's skin has not developed the horny layer which provides the impermeability characteristic of adult skin. The rate of diffusion of a gas through a permeable membrane is inversely proportional to the square root of its molecular weight. The relative rates of diffusion of phosphine and arsine compared with stibine = 1 are shown in the table. It will be seen that the diffusion rate of phosphine is 1.85 times that of stibine; and as a consequence phosphine is more likely to diffuse through skin into the bloodstream.

This rate of diffusion is also greatly influenced by residues of synthetic anionic detergents and/or quaternary ammonium (cationic) detergents. It has been shown that the rate of diffusion of a substance through a baby's skin can be increased up to 50 times by trace amounts of these detergents on the skin of baby. This is one reason why baby laundry should be washed in soap rather than detergent; that fabric softeners should not be used; and that soap rather than shampoo should be used for washing a baby's hair.

Very soon after the screening of the *Cook Report* programmes in late 1994, tests on post-mortem tissue samples were carried out by Professor Gordon Fell (a member of the Limerick Committee) on behalf of the Scottish Cot Death Trust to determine antimony concentrations in the livers of cot death babies as compared with babies which had died of other causes. The results were published in *The Lancet* on 22 April 1995.

It will be recalled that tests of this nature formed the basis of the first *Cook Report* programme. The *Cook Report* tests had demonstrated a wide variation in the incidence of antimony in the livers of cot death *versus* non-cot death babies. Of the liver samples from the 15 non-cot death babies, 14 did not contain any detectable antimony and one contained 1ng/g. Of the liver samples from the 40 cot death babies, 22 contained antimony in varying quantities and 18 did not contain any detectable antimony. It was noticeable, however, that there was a very wide variation in the concentrations of antimony within the 22 positive results: these varied from 0.90ng/g to 111ng/g.

Professor Fell's paper reported only the average results obtained from 25 cot death babies and 25 non-cot death babies. These were respectively 6ng/g and 7ng/g.

The paper stated that at least 16 of the 25 cot death babies had been sleeping on PVC-covered mattresses but no data was provided as to the amount of antimony in any of these mattresses. No information was quoted regarding the type of mattresses on which the non-cot death babies had slept.

On the basis of Professor Fell's averages, the Scottish Cot Death Trust issued a press release stating that raised levels of antimony in liver tissue are not linked to cot death.

In relation to the Fell study three points arise:

First, averages in this context are not helpful. For example, the average antimony level in the *Cook Report* cot death babies was 4ng/g but several contained very much higher levels. For the paper to have any real value, the figure for each cot death baby should be quoted.

It is known that the presence of antimony in the liver is primarily a measure of chronic exposure to antimony, but probably would not reflect an acute (lethal) dose. It follows that an average figure for antimony across a number of samples does not necessarily reflect lethal doses received by individual babies.

Secondly, Professor Fell's figure of 7ng/g for non-cot death babies is at variance with the known background level for babies, which is about 0.3ng/g. Clearly, therefore, a considerable number of both the cot death and non-cot death babies in Professor Fell's study had been subject to chronic (but not lethal) exposure to antimony. They certainly did not reflect the normal background level. (The *Cook Report* non-cot death babies did reflect the norm, with 14 of the 15 samples containing less than 0.5ng/g and one containing 1ng/g.)

Thirdly, it should be borne in mind that stibine is not the only poison which can arise from mattresses: any phosphorus present is a potential source of phosphine. According to the published results, Professor Fell did not analyse any of the 50 mattresses (25 cot death and 25 non-cot death) for phosphorus. Any number of the cot death babies in Professor Fell's study could have received sublethal doses of stibine but died from a lethal dose of phosphine or phosphine plus stibine. Significantly, at least 16 of the 25 cot death mattresses were known to have PVC covers and PVC frequently contains phosphorus in the form of both plasticisers and fire retardants.

Professor Fell's results as published in *The Lancet* are not meaningful; further, they are an example of the danger of incomplete study and reporting. They do not provide a scientific basis for the definitive statement which was issued by the Scottish Cot Death Trust.

In addition, two recent studies have attempted to replicate in the laboratory Richardson's generation of toxic gases by fungal activity.

The first of these was a trial commissioned by the Limerick Committee and carried out at the Public Health Laboratory in Bristol by Dr D. W. Warnock (a member of the Committee) and his associates. Using 23 PVC-covered mattresses on which babies had died of cot death, the team attempted to detect *S. brevicaulis* in the mattresses, but found that the micro-organisms present were a mixture of common *Bacillus* species. Using these species, they then attempted to generate toxic gases from antimony, arsenic or phosphorus present in the mattresses.

Samples from the mattresses were incubated and gases trapped on test papers containing silver nitrate and mercuric chloride. The exposed test papers were then tested for the presence of the elements antimony and arsenic.

Small positive results were obtained for antimony and arsenic in some of the tests. The antimony and arsenic could have been present on the test papers only as a result of transference in the gaseous phase.

Tests were not carried out for the presence of phosphorus, because phosphorus was already present in the test papers as an impurity.

In a summary of their paper, as published in *The Lancet* in December 1995, the authors stated:

> Our findings do not support the hypothesis that toxic gases derived from antimony, arsenic or phosphorus are a cause of sudden infant death. More sulphur was found in test papers exposed in plates containing bacterial growth than in those without such growth. This result suggests that the test paper reactions were due to the generation of sulphur-containing compounds during bacterial growth on the agar medium.

Two matters arising in these trials call the results into question. Each one is referred to in the *Lancet* summary just quoted.

The first relates to the micro-organism used in the testing programme. Warnock's paper makes it quite clear that he considered that the organisms which he found in the mattresses were all species of *Bacillus*, that is to say, bacteria. In this identification he may have been in error; what he described as *Bacillus subtilis* could have been *S. brevicaulis* (not a bacillus but a fungus) in its slime form.

Richardson had noticed some years previously that *S. brevicaulis* is dimorphic, that is, it can exist in two quite different forms. The first of these is the filamentous form, where the hyphae extend from the organism and the spores from the organism grow on the hyphae. The second is a gelatinous or 'slime' form, which bears no visible resemblance to the filamentous form. The second form, however, bears a very strong resemblance to *B. subtilis* (in fact, it may be that *S. brevicaulis* in its slime form and *B. subtilis* are one and the same).

Richardson had employed this dimorphism as a means of

identifying *S. brevicaulis*. Having found the fungus in its filamentous form, he would then plate it onto a nitrogen-rich medium such as malt extract and soy flour agar. If the filamentous form developed into the slime form, it was a very reliable indication that the organism was, in fact, *S. brevicaulis*. He would then use the filamentous form on mattress materials for his gas generation tests.

S. brevicaulis grows in its slime form when it has ample supplies of organic nitrogen compounds as a food source. The culture medium used by Warnock comprised 5% malt agar supplemented with 5% soy flour. As a result of the high proportion of nitrogen, whichever organism Warnock used grew in its slime form.

If, in fact, Warnock was not using *S. brevicaulis*, this may be accounted for by the following: Warnock states that on receipt of the samples of PVC mattress cover, he cut the samples into 20mm squares, which he then 'surface sterilised'. If it was Warnock's intention to detect the organisms naturally present on a cot death mattress, one wonders why he first sterilised the samples. In any event, this action may have destroyed any *S. brevicaulis* originally present on the cot mattress cover samples.

Whatever may be the force of the above, Warnock unequivocally replicated the generation of stibine by the action of *S. brevicaulis* on a cot mattress containing antimony. According to his test results, he positively identified *S. brevicaulis* on one mattress; this mattress contained a high proportion of antimony; and it gave a positive result for the generation of stibine. This same mattress also contained a small concentration of arsenic (commonly present in antimony as an impurity); and it generated arsine as well.

The fact that these results were achieved on only one mattress out of 23 does not detract from the relevance of the results.

(The results from this mattress parallel the findings of the Turner Committee. They too found the generation of stibine and arsine by *S. brevicaulis* on mattress material but could not achieve it consistently.)

Apart from the result on this one mattress, Warnock reported almost nil generation of arsine and stibine from culture tests on cot mattress PVC known to contain both arsenic and antimony. This result is consistent with the activity of *S. brevicaulis* growing on a medium containing a high proportion of nitrogen and therefore exhibiting its slime form. The reason is that the fungus, having a more than adequate supply of protein material available from the culture medium, obtained its entire requirement of nitrogen from this source and consequently did not consume any (or consumed very little) of the compounds containing the other Group V/Vb elements phosphorus, arsenic and antimony. Thus arsine and stibine were not consistently generated. Warnock should certainly have been able to generate arsine consistently; this reaction had been proved over 100 years before. The fact that he could not do so suggests that he was not working with *S. brevicaulis*.

However, the test conditions employed by Warnock did not replicate those normally pertaining in a baby's cot.

Richardson had previously noted that when he found *S. brevicaulis* on a cot mattress, it was always in the filamentous form and never in the slime form. The fact that the fungus was in this form in turn demonstrated that there was insufficient nitrogenous material in the cot for the needs of the fungus, the only sources normally available being the baby's sweat and vomit and residues of certain laundry products.

Under these conditions of insufficient nitrogen for its requirements, the fungus attacked compounds of the other Group V/Vb elements and it then excreted these foreign elements as the respective gases, just as it excretes ammonia if it has an over-sufficiency of nitrogenous compounds.

In order, therefore, to replicate faithfully Richardson's findings, the tests must use a medium which is low in nitrogen and the micro-organism employed must be *S. brevicaulis*, which in such a medium should then grow in its filamentous form.

Furthermore, if Warnock was correct in his identification of the organisms as *Bacillus* spp., then his whole investigation was pointless in any event, since there is no record of the generation of the trihydride gases of phosphorus, arsenic or antimony by bacilli.

The second matter arising from the Warnock trials relates to the presence of sulphur compounds in the culture medium, as evidenced by the copious generation of hydrogen sulphide from the cultures.

Richardson's method for the detection of the toxic gases was to absorb them in test papers containing metallic salts (silver nitrate and mercuric bromide) which combine with the gases, resulting in colour changes. The different combinations of colours indicated whether the gases detected were phosphine, arsine and/or stibine.

This test was derived from a very old-established classical method for the determination of arsenic, known as the Gutzeit test. This test depends on the reduction of arsenic compounds to arsine by zinc and hydrochloric acid. Any arsine formed is then detected by the change in colour of test paper impregnated with mercuric bromide, a yellow or brown-coloured adduct being formed.

Gutzeit recognised, however, that the presence of sulphur in the test solution would interfere, because the reducing agent would reduce any sulphur to hydrogen sulphide, which would also react with mercuric bromide to form a coloured compound. He therefore caused the evolved gas to pass through a paper impregnated with lead acetate, which trapped the hydrogen sulphide as lead sulphide.

Gutzeit's reason for eliminating sulphide was that the colour developed by any hydrogen sulphide which was formed would interfere with the colour developed by arsine. Richardson was aware of the potential interference by hydrogen sulphide and regularly tested for this by including lead acetate-impregnated papers in the petri dishes, but he did not encounter any such interference. In any event, S. brevicaulis does not have the capacity to reduce sulphur compounds to hydrogen sulphide and sulphur is not a common element in cot mattresses. (It is worth noting that the Turner Committee also did not encounter interference by sulphur in its tests.)

Test papers of the type used by Richardson (silver nitrate and mercuric bromide) had a purpose additional to the simple development of colour. They formed a trap for any phosphine, arsine and stibine generated by the fungus from the cot mattress and could be subsequently analysed for the presence of phosphorus, arsenic and antimony by methods which were specific for these elements. Richardson did this, thereby demonstrating the presence of phosphorus and antimony in the gases evolved by the fungus on the mattresses. These elements could only have reached the test papers in the gaseous phase, thus confirming the generation of phosphine and stibine from the mattresses. (Arsenic was detected only once in any significant quantity by Richardson; it is rarely incorporated in cot mattresses. Where arsenic was detected in small quantity, it apparently arose as an impurity in antimony.)

Warnock was not able to replicate Richardson's generation of the gases from cot mattresses. Two reasons for this have already been described, namely, the wrong culture medium and the use of either *S. brevicaulis* in its slime form or of *Bacillus* spp.

There is a further reason. As mentioned above, Warnock reported the copious generation of hydrogen sulphide from the test culture. This demonstrated that his culture medium contained a significant amount of sulphur, which was being reduced to hydrogen sulphide by some micro-organism other than *S. brevicaulis*. The evidence for the generation of hydrogen sulphide was the development of intense dark brown or black stains on the silver nitrate test papers.

The significance of the presence of sulphur in Warnock's test medium is threefold:

First, for any of the trihydride gases to be trapped in the test papers it is essential that the test reagent, whether silver nitrate or mercuric bromide, be immediately accessible to the gas. In the papers these compounds are in their solid or crystalline form and the absorption of any of the trihydride gases of phosphorus, arsenic and antimony is a surface effect on the crystals of the test reagents.

Where, however, the presence of sulphur leads to the generation of hydrogen sulphide, this brings about an interference. Hydrogen sulphide forms very stable and insoluble compounds with both silver and mercury, and in the presence of hydrogen sulphide the crystals are quickly coated with silver sulphide (in the case of silver nitrate papers) or with either mercuric or mercurous sulphide (in the case of mercuric bromide papers). As a result the trihydrides of phosphorus, arsenic and antimony generated by the fungus will not be trapped by the silver or mercury and therefore will not be retained in the test papers. Their presence in the gaseous phase will not be recorded, even by the subsequent analysis of the test papers.

Secondly, hydrogen sulphide can result in a further interference. Warnock's paper reveals that arsenic was present in only three of the 23 mattresses tested, and then in only very small concentrations. From a practical point of view, he was testing for antimony in PVC cot mattress covers. Antimony is added to PVC as a fire retardant in the form of antimony trioxide. Various investigations have indicated that S. brevicaulis does not react readily with antimony in this inorganic form, possibly because of its very low solubility, but more probably because the antimony is not associated with any food source for the fungus.

Thirdly, hydrogen sulphide forms very insoluble compounds with arsenic and antimony and the presence of any sulphide in the test medium would render any arsenic or antimony unavailable to the fungus.

In summary, where the presence of sulphur in the culture medium interfered with the tests, Warnock's results are meaningless. Such sulphur contamination is a result of the particular test conditions. Richardson did not find sulphur in cot mattresses, and neither did the Turner Committee. To my knowledge, no-one has ever reported the smell of hydrogen sulphide around a cot death victim; yet this is one gas which most people can recognise at very low concentrations.

It is known that PVC undergoes some degradation with age: it de-polymerises and liberates vinyl chloride monomer, which hydrolyses to form hydrochloric acid and other chlorine compounds. To counteract this, metallic stabilisers such as lead or other stearates are added to PVC to absorb the reaction products from the degradation of the PVC. Antimony trioxide reacts in the same manner as such metallic stabilisers, combining with the degradation products of the PVC to form other complexes, one of which may be antimony oxychloride. These complexes appear to be more amenable to reaction with the fungus than antimony trioxide, thus increasing the likelihood of stibine generation in the case of old PVC.

It was regrettable that, based on Warnock's paper, the Limerick Committee issued its first interim report in December 1995, implying that the Richardson hypothesis could not be substantiated. It should be noted that this paper was subject to peer review, but it would seem that none of the reviewers noticed the above shortcomings; or if they did, they failed to realise their significance.

A further trial was carried out during 1995. It was commissioned by a legal firm, Leigh Day & Co of London, who had been engaged by a group of bereaved parents considering legal action for damages. The study was carried out by Dr M. E. Callow and his associates at the School of Biological Sciences at the University of Birmingham.

The purpose of this study was, again, to test for the generation of (primarily) stibine by the action of *S. brevicaulis* on two compounds of antimony, the compounds selected being antimony trioxide, which is insoluble in water, and potassium antimonyl tartrate, which is fairly soluble.

The Birmingham study used several pure cultures of fungus, including two strains of *S. brevicaulis*, to check whether arsenic and antimony 'spikes' resulted in volatile arsenic and antimony compounds which would then be absorbed in silver nitrate test papers. The test papers were then analysed for the presence of arsenic and antimony by atomic absorption spectroscopy. For whatever reason, the papers were also analysed for phosphorus.

- All tests using arsenic spikes gave positive results.

- Tests using antimony trioxide spikes gave both positive and negative results, but mostly the latter.

- Tests using potassium antimonyl tartrate gave negative results.

The study reported that 'no evidence was obtained for the volatilisation of antimony compounds by any of the fungal isolates tested'. This statement is not true. Three samples gave positive results significantly above the lower limit of detection, although most of the results were negative. The three positive results were evidence of volatilisation of antimony, but – as with Warnock and Turner previously – the technique gave inconsistent results.

The Birmingham study also confirmed the generation of phosphine from phosphorus in the culture medium. The phosphorus was not added to the medium deliberately; it was there as a normal component of the medium itself.

The Birmingham study has the following shortcomings:

First, the use of antimony trioxide as a source of antimony does not replicate the conditions in a mattress, for the reasons set out above. Furthermore, antimony trioxide is only very slightly soluble in water, especially at the approximately neutral pH which pertains in media used for culturing micro-organisms. Hence it is not readily available to the fungus and so conversion to stibine is minimal.

Secondly, potassium antimonyl tartrate (commonly known as tartar emetic) would be most unlikely to provide antimony in a form suitable for the generation of stibine by the fungus. Although this compound is fairly soluble in water, the antimony is locked into the antimonyl-tartrate anion and consequently does not exhibit the typical reactions of antimony. Again, this compound is quite different from the type of antimony compound which would exist in a PVC cot mattress. The fungus will consume organic complexes which in some manner replicate protein, where the antimony supplants nitrogen. The antimony contained in an antimonyl tartrate ion does not come anywhere near meeting this condition.

To summarise, the results obtained by Callow are inconclusive as regards antimony. The techniques were unreliable in that they gave inconsistent results. Following some positive results for the generation of stibine, further research should have been carried out to determine the cause of this inconsistency.

'This is not to say, however, that Callow's results have no value – on the contrary. In addition to several instances of the generation of stibine, Callow demonstrated conclusively the generation of arsine and phosphine by fungi.

So far as Callow was concerned, the generation of phosphorus and arsine which he achieved was of no significance, as he was testing only for stibine. The results of his research, which had been commissioned to support a legal action based on the premise that stibine from mattresses had been the cause of cot death, were not nearly definitive enough for this purpose. At the time of writing, any legal actions of this type appear to be in abeyance.

From the point of view of the Richardson hypothesis, however, and particularly in the interests of eliminating cot death resulting from gaseous poisoning, Callow's research is of great importance.

So far as antimony is concerned, the danger arising from this element has largely been eliminated by the British cot mattress manufacturers themselves, who are understood to have discontinued the use of antimony in their products. In New Zealand antimony has never been knowingly incorporated in mattresses as a fire retardant, at least in recent times. Analysis of some cot mattress material has demonstrated that antimony is present, but at lower concentrations than were employed for fire-retardant purposes in Britain. In New Zealand the main source of deliberately incorporated antimony is polyester, in which it is used as a catalyst.

So far as arsine is concerned, Callow's work is of importance, especially in New Zealand and any other countries where the use of sheepfleeces for baby mattresses is common practice. All

Callow's experiments with arsenic demonstrated that arsine was generated, confirming yet again the finding which was first noticed in the 1820s.

Of even more importance is Callow's work regarding phosphorus. Phosphorus is commonly used in cot mattress fabrics in New Zealand, Britain and (presumably) many other countries. While the generation of ammonia from nitrogen and arsine from arsenic had been well established, there were relatively few references to the generation of phosphine from phosphorus.

Callow's report stated that the findings in relation to phosphorus were irrelevant and should be ignored. In his report he did not give any reason for this statement, but I subsequently ascertained that it arose from a comment made to him by the analytical chemist, Mr Ron Rooney. The reason Rooney advised Callow to ignore the phosphorus results was because the culture medium itself contained phosphorus and therefore the results could not be used in the proposed legal claim. From this perspective, of course, Rooney and Callow were correct; but in the broader context of the validity or otherwise of the Richardson hypothesis the phosphorus results were of crucial importance.

Phosphorus was found in Callow's test papers and its source could only have been the phosphorus in the culture medium. But equally, there was only one mechanism whereby the phosphorus was transferred from the medium to the test paper, and that was in the form of phosphine. Callow had therefore inadvertently but conclusively shown that phosphine is readily generated by microbiological activity from phosphorus compounds.

In conclusion, therefore, Callow's research is of prime importance: it replicates Richardson's findings, conclusively insofar as phosphine and arsine are concerned, and intermittently and partially in relation to stibine.

The intermittent generation of stibine achieved by Turner and Callow and the nil response obtained by Warnock may also have been caused by the use of a culture medium which was buffered to within the normal range of pH7.0 to pH7.5. Stibine (and arsine and phosphine) are similar to ammonia in that they all form a cation in solution, for example, the ammonium ion (NH_4^+) from ammonia. Likewise, stibine forms the stibonium ion (SbH_4^+). All these ions will form salts in solutions with a pH less than their pKb value, and consequently the gases are not readily liberated. It is possible that the generation of stibine as a gas will occur only from a substrate with a pH greater than that of a dilute solution of the hydroxide. Most micro-organisms will not flourish at high pH but Richardson has demonstrated that *S. brevicaulis* does so up to a pH of about 11.5. He has also demonstrated that cultures at high pH, spiked with antimony trioxide, appear to give consistent generation of stibine. It seems that the matter of pH is important in obtaining consistent generation of stibine.

In a baby's cot relatively high pH values can pertain, owing to the conversion of urea into ammonia. Another source of alkali is residues of soap, detergents, phosphate additives and fabric softeners. Any water in a baby's cot is probably not highly buffered, and consequently pH values capable of liberating stibine could sometimes be achieved.

Overall, there is clearly something which we do not understand about the bioconversion of compounds of antimony and phosphorus into stibine and phosphine respectively. That it occurs under certain circumstances is beyond question; but what those circumstances are remains unknown. This would be a fertile area for research and it is to be hoped that this challenge will be taken up. It will not now have any marked effect on the rate of cot death, but as a piece of technology it should be cleared up.

In the meantime, however, regardless of vagaries in their science and reporting by Turner, Warnock, Callow, and the Limerick Committee, it is beyond question that Richardson's findings have been replicated.

As regards the Report of the Turner Committee, the following reasons for the inconsistent results are now apparent:

First, large containers and detection papers were used to collect the gases, causing loss of sensitivity by dilution and the loss of the unstable gases through oxidation. As a result, there was little or no reaction with the reagent in the test papers, leading to negative test results for gas generation.

Secondly, as with Warnock's testing, the Turner Committee used a nitrogen-rich culture medium which did not encourage the formation by the fungus of the trihydride gases.

Thirdly, as with the testing by Warnock and Callow, the question of the pH of the buffered culture medium arises.

To summarise, the following results have been obtained since 1989 from testing for the generation of the trihydride gases phosphine, arsine and stibine and/or their alkyl homologues by *S. brevicaulis* and possibly related fungi from cot mattresses and/or spiked samples:

- Richardson obtained consistent generation of phosphine, arsine and stibine.

- Rooney demonstrated the presence of antimony in test papers developed by Richardson.

- The Turner Committee obtained generation of stibine and arsine, but not phosphine.

- Callow and associates obtained consistent generation of both phosphine and arsine.

- Warnock and associates achieved generation of stibine and arsine on one occasion.

The Richardson hypothesis provides an explanation for the extraordinary results achieved in Southland, New Zealand (see graph on page 22), where, following advice to discontinue the use of all chemical products in babycare, the cot death rate fell abruptly from a 3-year average (1986, 1987 and 1988) of 8.5 deaths per 1000 live births to 2.8/1000 during 1989. Significant reductions also occurred that same year in Otago and Canterbury, where the recommendation received some publicity, but the rate rose in the remainder of New Zealand (notably Auckland), where the news media ignored the research.

In essence, the advice to avoid chemical products covered chemical sterilants for clothing and bedding, chemical sterilants for feeder bottles and teats, synthetic detergents of all types, and fabric softeners. Parents were advised to use soap for all babycare washing and laundry purposes and to sterilise feeder bottles and teats by boiling them in water.

The fall in the cot death rate can be ascribed to the following two factors:

First, some synthetic detergents and all fabric softeners contain organically bound nitrogen compounds, such as dodecylbenzene sulphonic acid neutralised with some amine (for detergency); and long chain fatty acid alkylolamides (as foam stabilisers).

Furthermore, fabric softeners, which are based on quaternary ammonium compounds, are cationic detergents, and they function by reacting with residues in bedding and clothing left behind by the initial (anionic) detergent. The resultant 'salt' formed by this cationic/anionic reaction is insoluble, and so accumulates in fabric. It thus becomes a source of organically bound nitrogen.

Soap, by comparison, does not contain nitrogen. Therefore, by denying micro-organisms nitrogenous food sources, the growth of any fungus present, together with consequent generation of phosphine, arsine and stibine, was substantially impeded.

Secondly, many synthetic detergents contain phosphate additives, such as sodium tripolyphosphate and sodium hexametaphosphate, incorporated as builders and sequestrants. Phosphate compounds are precipitated in fabric by the action of hard water and can accumulate in bedding. Furthermore, the repeated use of detergents containing phosphate is known to result in accumulations of phosphate in fabric such as woollen blankets. Any residual phosphate in bedding would provide a food source to the fungus, from which phosphine could be generated.

Soap does not contain phosphate.

While I did not realise at the time why the dramatic Southland results had occurred, it is clear in retrospect that the above two factors are the probable cause of this reduction in cot death, and thus the results are entirely compatible with the Richardson hypothesis for the causation of cot death.

Further, it is possible that a third factor contributed to the reduction of cot death: the recommendation not to use chemical sterilants. All babycare chemical sterilants on the market – past and present – are based on strong oxidising agents, such as sodium perborate, sodium hypochlorite and chlorinated cyanuric acid.

Sodium perborate in solution generates hydrogen peroxide and can react to produce other peroxy- compounds. These are toxic in the body. They interfere with the clearance from the body of the oxidising substances produced during the progressive reduction of inhaled oxygen to water. The clearance of these oxidising substances is achieved by the glutathione peroxidase enzymes. If there is an additional loading of oxidising substances in the bloodstream as a result of absorption through the skin of hydrogen peroxide or related derivatives, the reducing capacity of the enzyme system becomes overloaded, resulting in generation in the body of the extremely damaging hydroxyl radical. This would adversely affect the health of a baby, rendering it more susceptible to cot death.

Chlorine-based oxidants such as hypochlorites and chlorinated cyanuric acid, when used for sterilising feeder bottles and teats, react differently from peroxy- compounds used in laundry products. Active chlorine from such chloro- compounds will react with many unsaturated organic compounds to form chlorinated derivatives. Chlorinated derivative compounds of this nature (such as dioxins, and chlorinated hydrocarbons such as chloroform) are now regarded with great concern as being extremely toxic and possibly having long-term health effects. One family of such compounds is known to have oestrogenic properties; other groupings are suspected carcinogens. If therefore, residues of chlorinated chemical sterilants used in babycare came in contact with the baby's food, some of the components of the food could be converted to a chloro-derivative. Again, it is axiomatic that any ingestion of chloro-compounds would adversely affect a baby's health.

13

Some Answers

The Richardson hypothesis was a revelation to me. It was the final piece of the jigsaw. I had realised in 1986 that cot death was caused by gaseous poisoning, but now the gases were identified. I had surmised that they were caused by microbiological activity, and now I knew what the fungus was. I had deduced that the gases acted on the baby's nervous system, and now I knew how. The hypothesis explained it all.

Nevertheless, to be valid the hypothesis had to fit every factor known about cot death, all the epidemiological observations. If there was a misfit, the hypothesis was thrown into doubt.

The way to test a theory is not to try to prove it – but instead try to *disprove* it. So I looked at what we knew about cot death and asked myself many questions, the same sort of questions as other people had posed over the years.

Why didn't we hear about cot death before the early 1950s?

Because until the 1950s it was quite rare, and in any event the deaths had sometimes been put down to other causes, such as respiratory failure. However, a steady increase in unexplained infant deaths had been noticed in Europe and North America in the early 1950s and was first described as a medical phenomenon by Dr A. M. Barrett in 1953. He estimated that unexplained infant deaths at that stage were three to four times what they had been a few years earlier. The term 'cot death' was coined to describe the sudden unexpected death of an apparently healthy baby while asleep.

By the end of the 1960s the consensus of scientific and

medical opinion was that this casualty rate was a new phenomenon, and in 1969 US paediatrician Dr J. B. Beckwith suggested the term 'Sudden Infant Death Syndrome' (SIDS) to describe the phenomenon. This description was introduced as code 798.0 in the 9th revision of the International Classification of Diseases in 1969 and the new item soon appeared in the mortality statistics of affected countries (demonstrating, incidentally, that cot death was a serious problem in some countries but very rare in others).

Cot death was rare prior to the 1950s because the use in mattresses of harmful materials containing phosphorus, arsenic and antimony had not really started. It was post-war technology which prompted the common use of phosphorus compounds as plasticisers and for other purposes, and (in some countries) arsenic as a preservative and antimony as a fire retardant. In addition, prior to the 1950s people used soap for baby laundry (detergents had not reached the domestic market), whereas they now use detergents and fabric softeners. These detergent substances contain organically bound nitrogen, which provides a food source for the fungus. Also some detergents contain phosphorus compounds which provide a source for the generation of phosphine.

If the chemicals have been in domestic use only since the 1950s, why were there some cot deaths before this time?

Because almost any source of phosphorus, arsenic or antimony will allow poisonous gas to be generated and these elements do occur naturally in some materials which historically have been used for babycare. Cot death was not common before the chemicals were deliberately introduced into mattresses, but it did sometimes occur because of these naturally present substances.

Sheep and goats ingest phosphorus, arsenic and antimony compounds from pastures and excrete them into their wool. Certain trees excrete these elements into their bark. Natural materials such as coconut fibre and kapok contain phosphorus and coconut fibre can also contain some arsenic. All of these natural products have been used historically in mattresses.

What about the claim that there is a reference in the Bible to a baby dying of cot death?

There is no such reference. Some people refer to the passage in the First Book of Kings, Chapter 3, starting at Verse 19. This is the well-known account generally referred to as 'The Judgement of Solomon', in which one mother's baby 'died in the night'. The passage goes on to say that '. . . [the mother] overlaid it.' So it was not a cot death.

Why have we not heard about the poisonous gas explanation before?

There is nothing new about it. In Europe in the 1880s many thousands of children died from the same cause, but in this case the poisonous gas was arsine (or trimethylarsine) produced by the same fungus from green pigments used in wallpaper, carpet and some furnishings. The explanation for these deaths was provided in 1892 by the Italian chemist Gosio and the gas was called 'Gosio's arsenic'.

There have been several similar instances since then of children being fatally poisoned, the last known case being in 1932, but this history seems to have been forgotten until Barry Richardson made the connection with babies' mattresses.

Even pathologists examining cot death babies seem never to have analysed body tissue samples for these toxic substances. Certainly in Britain it appears not one out of some 60,000 samples of post-mortem body tissue taken from cot death babies was ever analysed for phosphorus, arsenic or antimony.

Why do cot death babies show no symptoms?

Because the gas does not make them ill in the normal sense of the word. It acts by shutting down the nervous system, stopping heart function and breathing. But if the baby receives less than a lethal dose, its nerve functions continue more or less unaltered.

In some instances parents find their baby has stopped breathing through lack of heart function but is not dead. They pick it up and stimulate it, making it breathe again, and it recovers, apparently unaffected. This is called a 'near miss'. (Brain damage is a likely outcome of a near miss, due to oxygen starvation in the brain, but this would not be immediately apparent.)

Why aren't there many cot deaths among babies less than a month old?

Because it takes time for the fungus in a mattress to flourish and start generating gas. The fungus needs warmth and moisture and does not grow in a cool dry mattress, especially if there is no adequate source of nitrogen. However, very young babies can certainly die of cot death if placed on a mattress which has recently been used by an older baby and is already generating toxic gas.

Why aren't there many among babies over six months old?

Because the gas gives them a headache and they toss around, wake their parents and stand up in their cots. As a result they avoid continuing inhalation of the gas.

However, the risk extends beyond six months for babies suffering from any condition which reduces body weight and mobility. These babies are at risk for a longer period, typically up to about 14 months for premature and other underweight babies. Also, metabolic disorders increase the risk because they reduce the ability of the body to eliminate toxic substances.

Why do babies seem to be more at risk if births in a family are close together?

Because the fungus in the mattress from the previous use will be more readily viable in the case of the next baby, thus producing gas sooner.

Why has face-up sleeping saved so many babies' lives?

Because the toxic gases are all heavier than air (stibine, for example, is over four times heavier) and they flow away from the mattress down towards the floor. If the baby is face up, it is less likely to breathe them in.

The cot death rate has fallen for some years but is now levelling out. Why is it not continuing to fall?

Because face-up sleeping is only a partial solution. In certain circumstances it has only limited benefit:

First, it is not very effective against the danger of phosphine, because phosphine is only slightly more dense than air, and the warmth of the air around the baby will reduce this difference in density even more. This observation has been confirmed in Britain. The CESDI study in its first-year report demonstrated that face-up sleeping is not as effective against cot death as it was when first introduced in Britain. The same trend has been noted in New Zealand.

Secondly, face-up sleeping is not so effective when a baby is in a cot or bassinet with enclosed sides, because gases cannot flow away. The extra danger posed by enclosed cots and bassinets was recognised in Britain many years ago. Cots should have open sides to ensure good ventilation.

Does smoking cause cot death?

Smoking in itself does not cause cot death. If it did, cot death would have been identified as a serious problem well before the 1950s. For example, smoking was common in Britain during the 1930s and 1940s but cot death was not prevalent. Furthermore, smoking is very common in present day Japan and Russia but the cot death rates in those countries are minimal. Conversely, in the United States smoking is on the decline, yet cot death remains at a more or less constant level.

Nevertheless, a smoky environment may lead to underweight babies and may also weaken them, making them more susceptible to gaseous poisoning. The toxic dose of the gas is reduced if a baby is weak or underweight.

It is known that in New Zealand about 33% of all women

smoke during pregnancy, the figures for non-Maori and Maori women being 24% and 65% respectively.

No explanation for the apparent link between smoking and cot death has been advanced but I believe that the following may be an explanation: wafting cigarette smoke contains the element cadmium, which combines very strongly with the selenium in the vital glutathione enzymes, thus inactivating some of the enzymes and impairing the baby's health.

It should be noted, however, that smoking as a risk factor may simply be a parallel observation to the increased risk of cot death among lower socio-economic groups. That is, cot death is more prevalent among poorer families; and so is smoking. There may, in fact, be no causal association.

Why did your recommendations about going 'back to basics' in babycare lead to a reduction in cot death in Southland, Christchurch and Dunedin?

'Back to basics' meant:
- no synthetic detergents or fabric softeners; rather, all clothes and bedding were to be laundered using soap
- no chemical sterilants for nappies or bedding; rather, they were to be washed in soap
- no chemical sterilants for bottles or teats; instead they were to be sterilised in boiling water.

This had three effects. It eliminated:
- synthetic nitrogenous compounds from the baby's cot
- phosphate detergent residues from the cot
- chlorine contamination of the baby's bottle, food and teat.

It is not surprising that 'back to basics' reduced cot death, since it:
- denied the fungus an important food source
- removed a readily available source of phosphine from the cot
- removed from the baby's food a source of chloro- compounds which might adversely affect its health.

In Cot Death Association parlance, what I had discovered in Southland was another 'risk factor': the use of certain chemical products in babycare.

In 1995 the New Zealand Cot Death Study Group published an article saying that the use of nappy sterilants was not a cot death risk factor. They had questioned cot death and non-cot death families on the type of nappies they used, whether they soaked them before washing and how they washed them.

The article, which received wide publicity, stated that 'nappy cleaning methods are not related to SIDS' and that sterilant use as a major risk factor was refuted. Actually, this was not true.

The study demonstrated that babies were less at risk if nappy sterilants were not used. It also showed that the safest combination for cleaning nappies was to soak them in water and then wash them with soap, just as I had advised parents to do in Southland. Relative to other washing practices, this combination reduced the risk of cot death by at least 30%.

Why are bottle-fed babies more at risk than breastfed babies?

Whether bottle-fed babies are more at risk is far from clear. Breastfeeding is much less common in Britain (where about 24% of babies are breastfed) than in New Zealand (about 65% breastfed), yet the incidence of cot death is much lower in Britain than in New Zealand. These statistics contradict the proposition that bottle-fed babies are more at risk.

Certainly hypochlorite chemical sterilants, which are in common use in New Zealand and Australia, can remain in bottles and on teats if they are not rinsed. In New Zealand and Australia there is a specific instruction not to rinse bottles and teats after soaking. Thus the baby's milk can be contaminated with chloro-compounds, which are then ingested; and the baby can also ingest hypochlorite direct from the teat.

It is noteworthy that in Britain and elsewhere in Europe the instructions are quite different: rinsing after soaking is directed.

The adverse health effects of these chloro- compounds is well documented; they are certainly capable of weakening a baby.

COT DEATH RELATIVE RISK FROM VARIOUS LAUNDRY METHODS
FOR BABYWEAR AND COT BEDDING: NEW ZEALAND, 1987–1990

Relative risk of cot death (water/soap = 1)

2.0 1.5 1.0 0.5 0.0

Soak: Water   Water   Sterilant   None   Sterilant
Wash: Soap   Detergent   Rinse only   Detergent   Soap

Data: New Zealand Cot Death Study

COT DEATH RELATIVE RISK FROM VARIOUS LAUNDRY METHODS FOR BABYWEAR AND COT BEDDING: NEW ZEALAND, 1987–1990

This section of the study covered 323 cot deaths and 1360 'controls' (babies in households which had not suffered a cot death).

It shows that the risk of cot death was least when baby laundry was soaked in water only, followed by washing with soap rather than synthetic detergent.

This was the procedure recommended in the Southland trial.

Despite these figures, which indicated that the use of a nappy sterilant increased the risk of cot death by over 40%, the authors of the New Zealand Cot Death Study stated that the use or non-use of nappy sterilants made no difference to the risk of cot death.

Any baby in a weakened condition is more at risk from the toxic gases because the lethal dose is reduced.

Why does overheating a baby (say, through overwrapping) appear to cause cot death?

The extra warmth causes the fungus to increase gas generation markedly. A rise in body temperature from 37°C to 40°C causes gas generation to increase tenfold or more.

Many cot death babies are found with bedclothes over their heads. Has this caused the cot death?

Some 25% of cot death babies are found with bedclothes over their heads. This could lead to overheating, but would also result in lack of ventilation, trapping the toxic gases.

Why is cot death more prevalent in winter?

Because babies are wrapped up more and ventilation is less. Furthermore, if bedroom windows are closed, draughts which would cause the gas to dissipate are reduced or eliminated.

Why do more boys than girls die of cot death?

This has been attributed to the fact that boys have a higher metabolic rate than girls, and thus their body temperature can be somewhat higher. The rate of gas generation by the fungus increases rapidly with increasing temperature.

Many cot death babies have had minor illnesses (e.g. colds) before they died. Has the illness caused the cot death?

No. The infection has caused the baby's temperature to rise (e.g. a cold leading to a fever), thus heating the mattress more than normal, and the rate of gas generation has therefore increased.

Autopsies have shown that cot death babies frequently have bacterial and fungal infections in their throats and lungs. Why is this so?

If conditions in a baby's mattress have favoured the growth of the fungus *Scopulariopsis brevicaulis*, these conditions will also have favoured the growth of other micro-organisms which the baby has then breathed in. Many of these will have been harmless but they would still be noticeable at autopsy.

Why are re-used mattresses more dangerous than new mattresses?

Because the fungus has had a chance to establish itself in the mattress while the previous child or children slept on it. Then, when another baby uses it, the fungus is soon active and generates enough gas to poison that baby.

New mattresses are safer then re-used ones, but even new mattresses can generate the gases if they contain the harmful chemicals and the fungus has had time to develop.

Would the danger be eliminated if the mattress were cleaned?

No. Neither cleaning nor normal disinfectants will control infection by the fungus. Nevertheless, it is much less active when the mattress is very dry, so the old-fashioned practice of frequently airing a mattress (in the sunshine if possible) was a sound one.

Why does the cot death rate increase so markedly from the first baby in a family to the second, and from the second to the third, and so on?

First babies in a family frequently sleep on a new mattress, but parents tend to re-use the same mattress for subsequent babies.

Why is the cot death rate so high among Maori babies?

Cot death has a strong socio-economic bias, and less well-off parents cannot afford new mattresses. Many Maori people are in lower socio-economic groups and tend to borrow or re-use mattresses.

In addition, studies have shown that there is a high incidence of smoking among Maori women, and, as mentioned above, smoking appears to be a cot death risk factor.

COT DEATH RATE BY SOCIAL CLASS: BRITAIN, 1992
ALL COT DEATHS: BRITAIN AND NEW ZEALAND, 1992

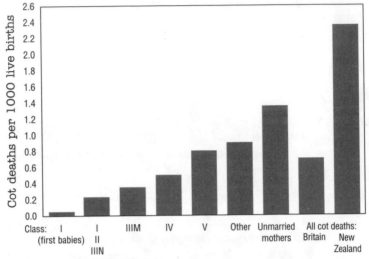

Data: Official British Statistics
New Zealand Public Health Commission

COT DEATH RATE BY SOCIO-ECONOMIC
STATUS: NEW ZEALAND, 1987–1990

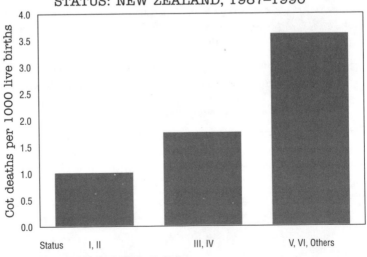

Data: New Zealand Cot Death Study

Cot Death Rate by Social Class: Britain, 1992
All Cot Deaths: Britain and New Zealand, 1992

This graph exhibits the very strong socio-economic bias in the incidence of cot death in Britain. The overall cot death rates for Britain and New Zealand are also shown.

Note the extremely low British rate for first babies within marriage of more wealthy parents (0.05/1000, only one baby in 20,000 births).

However, the cot death rate for wealthier parents increases with successive babies, reaching to about the average British level in the case of their third and later babies. The reason is that whereas the first baby almost certainly had a new mattress, this mattress was probably re-used for later babies.

Note the high rate for 'OTHER', believed to be mainly parents in the armed services living on service compounds in Britain and overseas. Re-use of issue mattresses is very common in these circumstances.

Social Classes (relates to occupation of father):

I	Professional
II	Managerial and senior administration
IIIN	Skilled occupations (non-manual)
IIIM	Skilled occupations (manual)
IV	Partly skilled occupations
V	Unskilled occupations
OTHER	Armed services, students, others not described

Cot Death Rate by Socio-Economic Status:
New Zealand, 1987–1990

As with the corresponding graph of British statistics, the strong socio-economic bias in cot death in New Zealand is evident. Less well-off parents who cannot afford new cot mattresses frequently borrow or buy second-hand mattresses.

In the past some observers have attributed the higher cot death rate among lower socio-economic groups in New Zealand to lack of parenting skills, but this is unjustified.

More recently, in an endeavour to explain the continuing high Maori cot death rate, some have pointed to perceived difficulties in communicating information about risk factors. The problem, however, is clearly not one of communication: for example, it is evident from the statistics that face-up sleeping has been widely adopted by Maori parents. Rather, so-called risk factors are ignored if they are regarded as unacceptable because of habit (e.g. smoking) or culture (e.g. bed-sharing).

The answer, therefore, is not to change communication style, but to communicate the right message – one which does not simply state risk factors but which provides a simple and inexpensive solution to cot death: to wrap mattresses in polythene sheeting.

Why is the cot death rate so high among unmarried mothers?

Again, because they are frequently not very well off and cannot afford new mattresses.

Why do wealthier parents almost never lose their first baby through cot death?

Because almost invariably they buy a new mattress for their first baby. It takes a while for the fungus to develop on a new mattress and start generating gases, by which time the baby is past the greatest at-risk age.

It has been noticed in Britain that if wealthier parents suffer a cot death, it is usually their third or later baby which dies.

Why does bed-sharing seem to contribute to cot death?

Because the gases can be generated in *any* bed, parents' included. (An adult is not greatly at risk if the gases are generated from a mattress. An adult's face is further from the mattress than that of a baby, and an adult exposed to the gas initially gets a headache and will take action well before the effects become more serious.)

It seems from the statistics that bed-sharing is a greater hazard if parents smoke than if they don't smoke. This statistical finding is consistent with the toxic gas theory. As mentioned above, a smoky environment can weaken a baby and thus increase its susceptibility to poisoning by toxic gases emanating from the mattress.

Are mattresses made from natural products safe?

In most cases, no. The only natural fibres known to be free of the harmful elements are cotton and silk, and even cotton is suspect because of additives frequently incorporated in cotton fabric.

Other natural products commonly used in mattresses include coconut fibre, horsehair, kapok and bark from certain trees. Being of natural origin, these products reflect the mineral composition of the land or pasture where they grow.

Phosphorus is normally present in sheepfleeces, and always present if the sheep have grazed on phosphate-fertilised pasture.

COT DEATH RELATIVE RISK ON VARIOUS MATTRESS
TYPES: NEW ZEALAND, 1987–1990

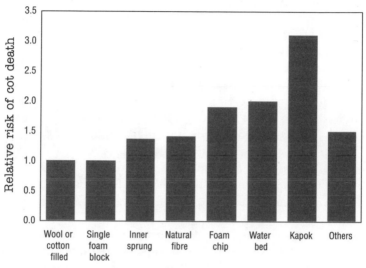

Data: New Zealand Cot Death Study

This graph shows that the risk of cot death is lowest on mattresses described as wool/cotton filled and that New Zealand-made foam block is equally safe. All other natural fibres, re-manufactured foam chip, and water-bed mattresses result in greater risk. The increased risk from inner sprung mattresses probably arises from the wadding (sometimes coconut fibre) or the fabric coverings of these mattresses.

Note the high risk associated with kapok, due to the very high phosphorus content of this fibre. Coconut fibre has shown a similarly high phosphorus content.

Water beds are not suitable for babies because their coverings may contain phosphorus. In addition, water beds are frequently kept heated, thus encouraging the growth of fungus.

Fleeces can also contain arsenic and antimony if the sheep have grazed on soil containing these elements. In New Zealand this appears to be common because of the volcanic nature of the soil in some areas. In Britain it was found that wool from areas in Cornwall near old tin mines readily produced arsine (arsenic is a byproduct of tin mining). By contrast, wool from chalkland pastures in Hampshire and Wiltshire does not contain arsenic, as it is not present in the soil.

Any animal ingesting phosphorus, arsenic or antimony excretes a proportion into hide or hair. Thus goatskins, horsehair and the like would potentially contain the elements.

Similarly, trees accumulate extraneous elements from the soil and excrete them through their bark. Ti-tree bark from Australia, coconut fibre and kapok have all been found to contain high concentrations of phosphorus, and sometimes arsenic and antimony.

It is not surprising, therefore, that an Australian study found that while babies on synthetic mattresses were three times more at risk of cot death if they slept face down, those on natural fibre mattresses were 20 times more at risk if they slept face down. ('Natural fibre' in this study referred to ti-tree bark and kapok, both enclosed in a permeable cotton mattress cover.)

The CESDI study in Britain has suggested that PVC-covered mattresses reduce the risk of cot death. Could this be true?

Certainly. Provided the PVC does not contain phosphorus, arsenic or antimony, PVC is the best material for covering a cot mattress. It has been found that babies are safer and healthier if they sleep on a mattress with a cover which is smooth and non-absorbent and thus can be easily and frequently cleaned.

The vented and open-weave mattresses currently fashionable were introduced because it was believed that cot death was caused by suffocation and therefore such mattresses would allow a face-down baby to breathe. In fact, accidental suffocation is extremely rare.

Vented and open-weave mattresses actually increase the risk

of cot death: they promote the growth of fungus and allow the toxic gases to reach the baby. They have a further health risk: dust mites infest the mattress, leading to asthma in children.

Why is the cot death rate lower among babies put to sleep on a wool 'waterproof' underblanket?

Waterproof blankets appear to be very effective in preventing moisture (for example, sweat) from passing to the mattress. The fungus will not grow under dry conditions and it is likely that waterproof underblankets reduce the risk of gas generation because of their water impermeability.

In New Zealand some blankets of this type are waterproofed by using a silicone or similar treatment. Any such treatment compound would be a good solvent for the toxic gases and would therefore tend to absorb gases being generated in the mattress.

Why is the rate of cot death in Japan so low?

There used to be virtually no cot deaths in Japan, although the rate is now rising slowly. The reason for the very low rate was that Japanese traditionally used untreated cotton futons for babies (and for adults as well). Cotton does not naturally contain phosphorus, arsenic or antimony.

Recently, however, as Japanese parents have started to adopt western babycare practices, mattresses, etc, the cot death rate in Japan has started to rise. It has been noted that when Japanese families emigrate to the United States their cot death rate rises to that of the local population.

Another reason for the low cot death rate in Japan is that fire retardants containing phosphorus and antimony are not used in mattresses there. If fire retardants are incorporated, they are usually compounds of boron, which do not generate any toxic gases.

Cot death is also virtually unknown in China, Thailand and Hong Kong, where cotton mattresses are normally used for babies.

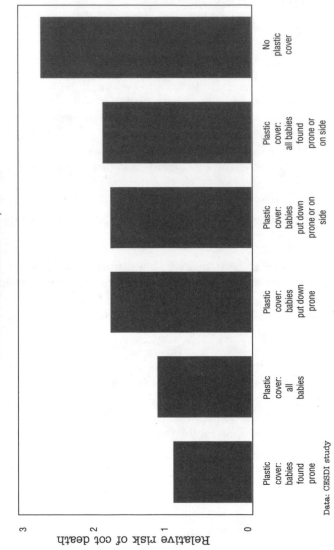

COT DEATH RELATIVE RISK ON DIFFERENT MATTRESS
COVERINGS: BRITAIN, 1993

Data: CESDI study

COT DEATH RELATIVE RISK ON DIFFERENT
MATTRESS COVERINGS: BRITAIN, 1993

This graph is based on information derived from the investigation of 101 cot deaths in three counties in Britain during the first year of the CESDI Study (1993). The crucial point arising from this data is that babies are less at risk if they are sleeping on a plastic-covered mattress: according to the figures, a baby sleeping on a fabric-covered mattress is about 2.5 times more at risk of cot death than a baby sleeping on a plastic-covered mattress.

The authors of the study interpreted this information to mean that the Richardson hypothesis was wrong, but they did not understand the significance of their findings. If a mattress has a plastic cover, the risk of poisoning arises from the cover only, and not from the mattress filling. Hence, if the plastic cover does not contain any of the harmful elements, it will not generate any of the toxic gases.

A fabric cover, by contrast, allows any gas from the mattress filling/s to reach the baby, as well as any gas from the cover itself. Furthermore, the conditions in a mattress filling (especially if the mattress is old) can be ideal for fungal growth; and if the cover is fabric, this growth will not be impeded.

Of course, all 101 babies had died, demonstrating that none of the mattress covers was safe; so the figures confirm the advice to wrap mattresses in polythene, or some other gas-impermeable sheeting free from the harmful chemicals.

Face-up sleeping led to a reduction in the cot death rate in New Zealand and Britain, but the rates then levelled off in both countries.

Most baby mattresses in Britain are PVC-covered, and now that antimony and (more recently) phosphorus have been removed from the plastic, the cot death rate can be expected to start falling again.

In New Zealand almost all mattress covers are non-plastic, and this certainly contributes to the very high cot death rate in that country. No further improvement can be expected in New Zealand until all the dangerous chemicals have been removed from mattress materials; or all mattresses are covered with polythene. The latter is the only immediate solution to cot death in New Zealand.

In summary, the CESDI study demonstrates beyond doubt that the safest mattress cover is smooth plastic; but (as the Richardson hypothesis demonstrates) the plastic must not contain phosphorus, arsenic or antimony.

Why is there virtually no cot death in Russia?

It has long been common practice in Russia to cover babies' mattresses with rubber sheeting. Like polythene, rubber is impermeable. This inhibits the growth of the fungus; and in addition any gas which is generated cannot reach the baby. Nor does rubber itself contain any of the harmful elements.

Moreover, it is common practice in Russia to use cotton mattresses for babies.

Why did so many babies of British Army personnel die of cot death?

For many years up to 1994 there was a high cot death rate among British Army families stationed on service compounds both in Britain and overseas. During 1986–1988 the cot death rate among Army personnel was 3.7 times that of the comparable civilian population. This high rate came about from two causes: the re-use of Army-issue mattresses; and the presence of arsenic in some mattress covers.

When service families required cot mattresses, these were on issue from the quartermaster and were returned when no longer needed. Thus there was multiple re-use, which led to increased likelihood of infestation with fungus.

Army mattresses were specially manufactured for their possible use in the tropics and consequently contained an arsenical biocide (OBPA). This biocide, a substituted arsine, is readily converted by *S. brevicaulis* into arsine itself or trimethylarsine.

Having been told by Barry Richardson of the danger from the biocide, in 1991 the Army withdrew these mattresses from service and discontinued the use of the biocide. (Regrettably, at least some of the replacement mattresses contained antimony.)

Is there a link between immunisation and cot death?

Whether there is a link has not been positively established, but anything which weakens a child makes it more susceptible to the poisonous gases, that is, the toxic dose is reduced. Immunisation causes an infection which affects some babies for a short time, so they could be more at risk during this period.

It appears from Australian research that a diet which is very high in vitamin C prevents cot death. Why would this be?

When the toxic gases are inhaled, they pass into the bloodstream and are converted into the corresponding ionic form of the gases. In the case of phosphine, for example, the phosphine molecule converts to the phosphonium ion. All of these ions are alkaline in reaction. If the baby has a high proportion of vitamin C (ascorbic acid) in its bloodstream, this will tend to make the blood slightly more acidic and absorb the alkaline ions in the form of the corresponding ascorbate salt. The ascorbate salt de-activates the toxic gas.

Why did people think that aspirin caused cot death?

Because people were in the habit of giving aspirin to their babies when they would not settle. In some instances the reason for the baby's agitation was that poisonous gas had given it a headache (a feature of poisoning by these gases). The aspirin drugged the baby to sleep, so it was then overcome by the gas.

What about the suggestion that cot death is caused by face-down babies running short of oxygen and rebreathing their own exhaled carbon dioxide gas?

The epidemiology and other known factors relating to cot death make it plain that this is not the cause. If it were:

- There would have been no sudden upsurge in cot death from the early 1950s onwards.

- Cot death would occur to an equal extent in all countries. (In fact, it is largely restricted to Western Europe, North America and Australasia.)

- There would be no difference in the cot death rate between first and later babies. (In fact, there is a marked difference, as shown in the graph on page 64.)

• The cot death rate would be the same across all socio-economic groups. (In fact, the rate varies widely, as shown in the graphs on page 140.)

This rebreathing concept emanates from the United States, where the use of PVC-covered mattresses containing antimony fire retardants and phosphorus-based compounds is very widespread. One peer-reviewed research paper propounding the concept suggested that the rebreathing of carbon dioxide applied especially when babies were sleeping on pillows filled with granulated polystyrene foam. That cot deaths occurred on such pillows is not surprising: polystyrene foam is extremely flammable and therefore frequently contains antimony- or phosphorus-based fire retardants.

The Richardson hypothesis has received scant attention in the United States. It is clear that the researchers are mistaking poisoning by phosphine and/or stibine for asphyxiation by carbon dioxide.

Why does the cot death rate appear to be lower among babies using a dummy?

There is a fairly obvious explanation for this. If a mother wishes the baby to keep a dummy in its mouth, she will not place it on the mattress face down. The likelihood is that the baby will be face up and therefore less at risk of gaseous poisoning.

Most cot death researchers claim there are many causes of cot death. Why do you say there is only one?

There is no evidence to support the claim that cot death is 'multifactorial', to quote the usual term. This idea seems to have been invented to explain why traditional researchers have not been able to solve the problem. They take the line that 'cot death is an extremely difficult problem because it has many causes'.

This is clearly not the case. The mode of cot death – apparent total lack of symptoms, no prior warning, and (until now) no discernible cause – is the same pattern wherever cot death occurs in any part of the world.

Added to this are the risk factors identified by epidemiology, which are the same wherever cot death is prevalent: face-down sleeping; overheating; underweight; birth prematurity; the at-risk age range; greater risk during winter; socio-economic disadvantage; higher incidence if parents smoke; higher rate among boys than girls; increasing risk for second and subsequent births in a family.

Other similarities include the fact that cot death was recognised as a phenomenon in the affected countries at the same time, the fact that it is prevalent only in western-style countries, the similarities noted in 'near miss' cases, and the similarity of after-death symptoms such as cyanosis and petechiae.

It is inconceivable that these identical features throughout all affected countries – with no points of difference – could result from a wide variety of causes. The totality of the evidence points towards there being one cause of cot death: gaseous poisoning.

What is the solution?

All sources of the elements phosphorus, arsenic and antimony should be excluded from the baby's environment. This applies especially to bassinet and cot mattresses, which should be subject to a strict specification in relation to these elements.

Until this can be achieved, babies must be protected against the risk of poisoning by covering cot mattresses with an impermeable material. The most convenient means is to wrap the mattress in heavy-grade clear polythene (not PVC), secured firmly beneath the mattress with strong adhesive tape but without making the polythene on the underside of the mattress airtight.

The New Zealand Cot Death Association has stated that mattress-wrapping may be dangerous for babies because of suffocation and overheating. Is this true?

No, provided that thick polythene (not PVC) is used and that it is firmly taped underneath the mattress. Mattress-wrapping has been widely publicised in Britain since 1989 and there has not been one recorded cot death on a polythene-wrapped mattress.

Accidental suffocation by babies is extremely rare. A noted feature of newborn babies is their ability from the time of birth to lift their heads from the prone position, which obviates any risk of suffocation. Furthermore, the CESDI study has shown that babies are safer and healthier if they sleep on mattresses which are covered with a smooth plastic surface. (Of course, this plastic must not contain any phosphorus, arsenic or antimony.)

Similarly, the claim about overheating has no justification. The heat insulation provided by the relatively thin layer of polythene is minimal compared with the heat insulation arising from any cot mattress. The polythene sheet should be covered with a fleecy underblanket (preferably cotton) and this will absorb any perspiration from the baby. In any event, the danger of cot death from overheating is the accelerated generation of the toxic gases. Since the polythene sheet stops the gases from reaching the baby, overheating as a risk factor becomes irrelevant.

14

When You Can't Answer, Fudge It

I f ever an organisation had an opportunity to be at the cutting edge of solving cot death, it was the New Zealand Cot Death Association. Blessed with a high public profile, the support of media personalities and public money seemingly on tap each annual appeal day, CDA could really make a difference. Instead they have lost the plot.

Any disinterested person hearing about my Southland research and the Richardson hypothesis would no doubt expect CDA to want – at the very least – to discuss them with me. But years of sending CDA letters, reports and published papers did not elicit a single reply until November 1995. In the late 1980s I had obtained an appointment to meet CDA's national co-ordinator, Dr Shirley Tonkin, but she stood me up.

Despite my efforts to engage them in debate, until May 1996 CDA would not discuss with me either the Richardson hypothesis or any of the scientific issues I raised with them. Their correspondence dealt only with matters of an administrative nature.

The New Zealand Cot Death Association has a number of branches around the country which co-ordinate support for bereaved parents, meetings and fundraising at the local level. I first came into contact with this organisation in 1986, when I launched my 'back to basics' campaign in Southland. I had decided to announce the campaign at a meeting of the Southland Cot Death Society, but in retrospect this move was a mistake: the local society was furious.

Over the years I have discovered an interesting feature about cot death societies, which applies not only in New Zealand. One of their stated functions is to provide a source of support and comfort for bereaved parents. It's a laudable purpose, but it also provides a means of ducking the issues. Using the line that 'we mustn't upset bereaved parents any more than they already have been', cot death societies – it seems to me – simply ignore or quash new ideas that don't 'fit' their current line. The rationale they put forward is that parents might blame themselves for the baby's death if they hear about a possible cause which they could have avoided.

And this was what I ran up against in Southland. If, indeed, going back to basics in laundering babies' clothes would reduce cot death – so the argument went – parents who had used these products and lost babies would suffer feelings of guilt.

But in Southland I discovered something else as well: the cot death societies might think this way, but the parents themselves most certainly don't. Bereaved parents are desperate to know why their baby has died, regardless of how the answer might make them feel. They are frequently suffering from feelings of guilt anyway, and not having an answer to their question doesn't remove those feelings. And these parents are usually very keen to have an answer for another reason as well: they don't want other parents to experience the grief of a cot death. During the years that I have been involved in cot death research, tearful bereaved mothers have urged me on numerous occasions to keep on searching for the cause. Not one has ever suggested that my research might be hurting parents – a far cry from the reaction I would encounter over the years from CDA.

I was to come up against this difference in agenda many times, but it didn't take long for the impact to be felt after I had announced my Southland research. My recommendations had also reached Christchurch and Dunedin (leading, incidentally, to reductions in the cot death rate in those areas as well as in Southland) and the *Christchurch Press* and *Christchurch Star* had both published an article giving details.

Felicity Price, then regional co-ordinator of the Canterbury Cot Death Association and herself a bereaved mother, is a well known media personality in the region, and she weighed in. According to her, the *Christchurch Star*, *Christchurch Press* and *Southland Times* had been unbalanced in their reporting of my research, and she laid complaints against all these newspapers with the New Zealand Press Council. Only one complaint was upheld, and that only in part (the Council agreed that the *Christchurch Star*'s reporting had been unbalanced) but it was a foretaste of the opposition I would encounter in my dealings with the cot death establishment.

In August 1995 I turned on Radio Pacific one afternoon to find Shirley Tonkin talking about the forthcoming Red Nose Day appeal. Radio Pacific, as a nationwide talkback station, encourages calls on controversial issues and I phoned in. To no avail: I was informed that Dr Tonkin had given instructions that I was not to be allowed to talk on the programme. I complained immediately to the station manager, Derek Lowe, but he backed her: since CDA had purchased the time slot (costing some thousands of dollars), they called the shots regarding who got to speak on air.

From a commercial standpoint, Derek Lowe was quite right. CDA had certainly bought the time. But CDA aren't a private organisation: they are funded by public money, and as such have a responsibility to publicise all relevant views, not just their own.

In the Autumn and Spring 1995 issues of their *Newsletter* items appeared on the Richardson hypothesis, both denying the validity of the research. In February 1996 I asked for the right of reply, again pointing out that CDA were a public body and could not simply do as they chose regarding publicity of views contrary to their own. CDA refused. One reason advanced was that they didn't want to upset bereaved parents by including in their *Newsletter* an item about an 'unproven' theory (even though they had now *twice* written about the theory in the *Newsletter*). At the time of writing (June 1996) I am still waiting for the right of reply.

While such matters as the publication of theories and the right of reply may be of particular concern to researchers and academics, other aspects of CDA's activities are of more concern to the general public.

In April 1996, in order to carry my research forward, I placed advertisements in several Auckland community newspapers, seeking mattresses on which babies had died of cot death. This immediately put me in contact with bereaved mothers.

Cot death mothers, of course, are found in all sectors of society, but they tend, from my observation, to have something in common: by and large they are thoughtful people with considered views. This isn't surprising: cot death is one of the most heartbreaking experiences a person can suffer and these mothers go through a lot of pain. They think long and hard about it and they ask a lot of questions. Right now some of them are asking questions about CDA.

They are the same sort of questions the media are starting to ask about CDA, such as 'Why, after all the research, don't we know the answer to cot death?' and 'Where does all the Red Nose Day money go?' and 'Why won't CDA publish the cot mattress theory and let parents decide for themselves?'

The answer to the first of these questions is a simple one: cot death researchers are almost exclusively medical people looking for a medical solution. But cot death is, by their own definition, not a medical problem in the first place; a baby's death is termed a cot death only if there is no apparent medical cause. Since cot death researchers have tended to think only along the lines of possible medical solutions, they have ignored environmental chemistry and the toxicology associated with it.

CDA state quite freely that they do not know the cause of cot death and this has been their standard line ever since their inception. Using this rationale CDA have focused on all sorts of so-called 'risk factors', chiefly face-down sleeping, smoking, bottle feeding and overheating – none of which are *causes* of cot death.

CDA still adhere to the 'multifactorial' theory – the idea that cot death has many causes. Yet they have never been able to suggest a single one; all they talk about is 'risk factors'. A good fudge. They seem to overlook the corollary arising from the multifactorial theory: if there were, say, ten different and identifiable causes of cot death, surely it would have been ten times as easy to find just one of them. But they admit themselves that they haven't found any.

Actually, CDA have been told the cause. They first heard about poisoning by microbiological activity in 1986 (from me) and they received full details of the Richardson hypothesis in 1991 (from Barry Richardson).

Certainly the general public believe that CDA don't know the cause of cot death – their response to appeals shows this. Red Nose Day, as it is known in New Zealand (and elsewhere), comes around each August and is accompanied by massive publicity. Television New Zealand throws its weight behind the campaign and the money usually pours in. In 1995 an estimated gross sum of $900,000 was donated.

But it is instructive to note where this money ends up. In 1995, for example, CDA's estimated receipts were $300,000. So where did the remaining $600,000 go? It is known that the National Child Health Research Foundation receives one quarter of the income – a point which is certainly not put before the New Zealand public, who believe they are donating specifically for cot death research. Television New Zealand receives between $100,000 and $200,000 each year for its participation in the appeal. And from these figures it would appear that a sizeable chunk also ends up in the hands of the public relations consultants who are associated with it. An apparent net result of 30-odd percent for cot death research is hardly what the donating public expects.

Questions are now being asked about what CDA do with their funds. Among the public there is a groundswell of impatience with the apparent lack of results. After all, New Zealand still has the highest cot death rate in the world (about 2.0 deaths per 1000 live births in 1992 and 2.1 in 1993) and the figures for the Maori community are appalling (6.9 for 1992, rising to 8.0 in 1993).

Not only among the public is there disquiet, but within CDA itself a policy conflict appears to be developing. The high cot death rate among the Maori community has attracted the attention of influential figures within its ranks. As a result, Maori cot death workers – among them a member of the CDA Board – are calling for CDA's resources to be directed specifically to the problem of Maori cot death. Given that CDA's advice to parents, which is limited to a few risk factors, does not seem to be having any impact on the Maori rate (a fact which some Maori attribute to communication style), this demand from Maori cot death workers does not seem unreasonable. After all, even the now defunct Public Health Commission, having stated in 1993 that it aimed to reduce the rate among Maori to 4.5/1000 by 1997 and to 2.5/1000 by the year 2000, subsequently admitted that it considered these objectives to be 'challenging'.

Shirley Tonkin apparently won't have a bar of this demand by Maori cot death workers. According to her, New Zealanders, being all one people, are all amenable to the same CDA strategy for reducing cot death. This is just one more fudge. It conceals a deeper split in basic philosophy about cot death: should CDA's resources go to the workers at the coalface or the researchers in the ivory towers?

No critique of CDA would be complete without mention of its apparent linchpin, Dr Ed Mitchell. Although not a member of the CDA board, his views hold tremendous sway. Ed Mitchell is an Associate Professor of Paediatrics at Auckland Medical School. He has published numerous papers on cot death over the years, but his main contribution to cot death research has been the New Zealand Cot Death Study, carried out over a period of three years from November 1987 to October 1990. The results of this study have formed the basis of CDA's advice to New Zealand parents for the best part of a decade.

Ed Mitchell is a first-class epidemiologist, and the New Zealand Cot Death Study reflected this forte. Epidemiology studies a problem by identifying and describing its outward manifestations. 'Cases' (instances where a problem has occurred) and 'controls' (where there has been no problem) are compared by examining the various features which are characteristic of each group. Similarities and differences are noted and used to identify contrasts which might account for the problem. Epidemiology is a widely used medical technique and has yielded valuable results. It did so in the case of the New Zealand Cot Death Study.

In this context, the 'cases' were cot death babies and the 'controls' were living babies. Obstetric records were examined and parents were asked a comprehensive range of questions about their babycare practices. The study confirmed, once and for all, that face-up sleeping reduces the risk of cot death. It threw up three other apparent risk factors: smoking by the mother, lack of breastfeeding, and babies sleeping with another person. According to Mitchell in 1992, these four factors could account for 82% of all cot deaths, though the paper was devoid of any explanation why the deaths occurred!

Mitchell and his co-workers described these four factors as 'modifiable' – things parents could do something about – and these four so-called 'risk factors' have formed the central thrust of CDA's advice to parents ever since. Not all these would be achieved readily: breaking smoking habits is notoriously difficult; not every mother can or wishes to breastfeed; and some cultures have a strong bias towards babies sleeping with their parents. But face-up sleeping could be adopted by parents immediately.

And it worked, at least among non-Maori people. The benefit of face-up sleeping had been receiving publicity in New Zealand from late 1989 and in July 1990 CDA launched their national cot death prevention programme, endorsing especially face-up sleeping. By 1992 the nationwide cot death rate was half the 1989 figure.

But no one – not CDA, nor Ed Mitchell, nor anyone else in New Zealand – could explain why face-up sleeping worked, and they still say that they can't explain it. What's more, Ed Mitchell says he isn't particularly interested in why it works. Neither, it would seem, are CDA. There is a corollary to this: not being able to explain why face-up sleeping works, CDA now can't explain why – even with the very wide acceptance of face-up sleeping – the cot death rate has levelled off.

Likewise, no explanation has ever been advanced by CDA for the remaining three 'modifiable risk factors', and two of these (breastfeeding and bed-sharing) are still the subject of controversy in any event.

For a time face-up sleeping caused a sharp drop in the rate of cot death. But then CDA were faced with something different: environmental science entered the picture, in the form of the Richardson hypothesis. Epidemiology had described just about everything that could be noted and described about cot death; and not surprisingly, some of these observations had pointed to actions which would reduce – indeed, had reduced – the rate of cot death. But now CDA were confronted with a proposition, from outside the field of medicine, which explained it all. And because it explained the cause, rather then merely describing the phenomenon, the solution to cot death became obvious.

Suddenly, it was a new ball game. Medical science had not uncovered – and, if the proposition was right, never would un-cover – either the cause of cot death or how to eliminate it. It was also a golden opportunity for CDA: they could have added the Richardson hypothesis to their store of knowledge, explained all their epidemiology and wrapped up the problem.

Instead, having met Barry Richardson during a visit to Britain in 1991, Shirley Tonkin summed up her reaction to his hypothesis in the *New Zealand Herald* in December of that year: 'This man has an idea. He has got no proof at all. Parents need not worry about it.' Just how she reached this conclusion has always escaped me. But CDA backed their national co-ordinator and set about contradicting the hypothesis.

There were several avenues CDA could follow to achieve this end: they could ignore it; they could say it wasn't 'proved' (not to their satisfaction, anyway); they could label it 'dangerous'; they could try to discredit anyone who publicised it; and they could say that even if it were correct, it wasn't applicable in New Zealand anyway.

They did the lot.

Out went the word from CDA that the Richardson hypothesis 'wasn't proved'. By this they meant that it had not been accepted by the medical profession because it hadn't been through the normal 'peer review' channels.

It is difficult for the lay person to realise how bogged down the medical profession is with the concept of peer review (the examination of research papers by other people in the same field). In the medical arena, peer review often takes over from common sense. For example, when Barry Richardson first approached FSID with his new hypothesis, the immediate reaction of Joyce Epstein was to reject it because it wasn't reported in the literature! How a new discovery could have previously been reported in the literature escaped Barry Richardson. (The names of Bell, Faraday, Rutherford, Curie, Semmelweiss and others come to mind: their discoveries had not been previously reported either!)

Just how medical people would review environmental chemistry, CDA didn't explain, but in any event CDA have a double standard when it comes to the proof they require for a proposition. CDA publish their advice regarding face-up sleeping and non-smoking based on the New Zealand Cot Death Study, which was peer-reviewed. However, since Ed Mitchell admits that he cannot explain why face-up sleeping has reduced cot death, presumably the reviewers were not concerned to understand the mechanism either.

By contrast, the Richardson hypothesis *does* explain the mechanism (as well as all the other epidemiological observations regarding cot death). Yet his research is either completely denied or rejected for 'lack of peer review'. (Actually it has been peer-reviewed and published in a very reputable journal.)

At least face-up sleeping produced a demonstrable result, but the same cannot be said for the non-smoking proposition. It too appeared in the peer-reviewed New Zealand Cot Death Study, and is trotted out by CDA as a 'modifiable risk factor', but the only evidence is the epidemiology. No one can point to a reduction in cot death as a result of non-smoking. Nor has the epidemiology been explained.

And yet it was all peer reviewed. Peer review starts to look like an old boys' network – convenient when you need it. But it can also be the blind leading the blind, and a good way of suppressing a new idea.

'Dangerous': the word is always a winner if you want to catch the attention of parents. This is Ed Mitchell's hobbyhorse and he has used it time and again. He talks about the possibility of babies suffocating if parents wrap their mattresses in polythene; or that they might become overheated, or sweat. All of this completely ignores the total success of mattress-wrapping in Britain (not one reported cot death on a polythene-covered mattress in the last six years) and the incontrovertible finding by Peter Fleming in the British CESDI study that the best mattress cover for a baby is a smooth plastic film.

When logical arguments fail, some people resort to the fallback position of trying to discredit the messenger. In the May 1996 issue of *North & South* CDA Chairman Tim Burcher decided to take a swipe at my scientific credibility. Referring to the Southland research, he said: 'This is the same Dr Sprott who seven years ago equally vehemently held the view that . . . a product used to sterilise soiled nappies was the cause of the condition. New Zealand research showed it was not the cause.'

The implication was clear: that having been 'proved wrong' over Southland, I had now jumped onto another bandwagon – the Richardson hypothesis – and the latter would prove to be just as 'fallacious' as the former.

I feel some sympathy for Tim Burcher. He is a very likeable fellow, a partner in the Auckland law firm of Short & Co. But I concluded that he was clearly not aware of the facts. My recommendations in Southland were a 'back to basics' package, involving all manner of modern proprietary products. The focus was never on one item; and furthermore, as explained in chapter 13, the New Zealand research which Tim Burcher relied upon didn't yield the conclusion Ed Mitchell claimed it did. (See graph on page 136.) Nevertheless CDA continue to repeat their line about the Southland research regardless. The fact that the region's cot death rate fell dramatically doesn't seem to figure with them. As has already been clarified (in chapters 12 and 13), the Southland results exposed a cot death 'risk factor' and are entirely consistent with the Richardson hypothesis.

Far more hazardous than sideswipes against my scientific credibility was CDA's knee-jerk response that even if the Richardson hypothesis was valid, it didn't apply in New Zealand anyway. No sooner had news of the *Cook Report* programmes reached this country, than Shirley Tonkin announced that New Zealand mattresses were manufactured differently and didn't contain any of the harmful antimony, and therefore the hypothesis was irrelevant here.

How did she know? You can't tell by looking at a mattress or by reading the component breakdown on a label. Even the mattress manufacturers are very unlikely to know the chemical composition of the materials (for example, foam, polyester fill and fabric) which they use. In the case of New Zealand mattresses, such materials are almost invariably imported, from many sources all over the world.

The only way to be sure that an element is not in a mattress is by chemical analysis of the various components which are present in that mattress. CDA had never done this, nor had the mattress manufacturers. Nor had any of the New Zealand distributors who were supplying the componentry to the manufacturers.

Shirley Tonkin got it wrong. Some New Zealand cot mattresses do contain antimony.

And she had also repeated the mistake made by FSID in Britain. She jumped on the antimony bandwagon, ignoring the danger posed by phosphorus and arsenic. However, virtually all New Zealand mattresses contain phosphorus, while some contain antimony as well as phosphorus.

It was a serious error on the part of CDA. Despite their insistence that New Zealand babies were safe from this gaseous poisoning, actually the babies were in just as much danger as British babies had been from stibine – even more so, because of the widespread incidence of phosphorus in New Zealand cot bedding.

CDA maintain a firmly closed mind, and in this they have plenty of company. FSID answers my correspondence but have been consistently critical of Barry Richardson and the hypothesis. The Scottish Cot Death Trust have been courteous and initially seemed interested in Richardson's work, but quickly changed their attitude, apparently at the urging of Professor Fell (who is a member of the Limerick Committee). Letters to the Irish Cot Death Association have been ignored. Since 1989 I have four times visited the Canadian Foundation For the Study of Infant Deaths, based in Toronto: the reception has been friendly but there has never been any real interest or follow-up. They take the same line regarding mattresses as CDA: that the hypothesis doesn't apply because the chemicals aren't used in Canada. (Actually, they are.) My efforts to contact cot death associations in Australia, both nationally and in various states, have elicited no reply. Likewise in the United States.

In early 1996, I offered to present a paper to the Fourth International SIDS Conference in Washington D.C. but this was declined.

I've come to the conclusion that Shirley Tonkin supports any publicity which denies the Richardson hypothesis. In March 1995 a BBC *QED* tele-vision programme, 'Cot Death', claimed to have overturned the findings of the *Cook Report* programmes. According to the programme:

- Testing of 19 cot mattresses had failed to reveal the presence of *Scopulariopsis brevicaulis*, except in two cases.

- Testing of PVC samples from the mattresses had failed to generate stibine (except for a small amount in two cases, which was attributed to contamination).

- *QED* showed a brief clip from an interview with Ron Rooney in which Rooney said that a black stain on test papers did not necessarily prove the presence of antimony. Rooney said, 'There are many different gases that cause these papers to darken.'

- The ongoing CESDI study showed that far from PVC being dangerous, babies were actually safer sleeping on PVC-covered mattresses; and that re-use of mattresses did not increase the risk of cot death.

Shirley Tonkin described it as a 'most excellent television documentary'. Actually:

- The microbiologist, Dr Jane Nicklin, was mistaken in her fungus identifications because she didn't realise that *S. brevicaulis* can exist in two forms.

- It is clear from their dark colour that the silver nitrate papers sent to the analyst, Dr Mike Thompson, were contaminated with sulphur (a problem described in Chapter 12).

- *QED* cut Ron Rooney's statement. His full statement was: 'There are many different gases that cause these papers to darken so I analysed the papers to confirm that antimony and phosphorus were present.' The editing reversed the meaning of what Rooney had actually said.

- *QED* also omitted to include a statement made to them by Ron Rooney that he had proved the presence of antimony in test papers previously supplied to him by Barry Richardson.

- As for black stains on test papers, Barry Richardson didn't get these. His papers turned either yellow for phosphine, or beige darkening to mauve for stibine. Mike Thompson's black-stained papers indicated faulty procedure and were not worth investigating; so it was pointless for *QED* even to ask Ron Rooney about the relevance of black stains. Anyone knowledgeable about such analyses would have been aware that the stains came from sulphide.

- The findings from the CESDI study as presented in the programme were misleading. Babies are indeed safer on a mattress with a smooth plastic cover; the danger arises if the plastic cover contains the harmful elements. So the issue isn't whether a mattress is or is not covered with PVC; it's whether or not the PVC contains the harmful elements.

- As for the risk from re-use of mattresses, the CESDI findings were at variance with official British statistics about the higher cot death rate among later babies.

The programme certainly didn't overturn the Richardson hypothesis – scientifically, I thought it was rubbish – yet it received an accolade from Shirley Tonkin.

If asked about the gaseous poisoning hypothesis, Shirley Tonkin replies that not only is it unproven, but it is likely to scare parents and distract them from taking the CDA precautions. According to her, a proper scientific trial could cost more than $300,000 and is beyond the resources of New Zealand researchers. To which I would answer: it shouldn't be beyond their resources – the public donates about $1,000,000 every year for cot death research. But even if it is too expensive, why don't they take notice of overseas research which has confirmed the hypothesis and, especially, take notice of the greatly reduced cot death rate in Britain?

But not everyone is listening to the CDA line, and even some in the cot death establishment seem to be breaking ranks.

Ed Mitchell springs to mind. Having described the Richardson hypothesis in December 1995 as 'a theory which has been totally discredited' (and myself as 'irresponsible' for advancing it), by February 1996 he was terming it 'interesting and plausible', and in March he thought there 'may be some justification for ongoing work on the Richardson hypothesis'.

In April 1996 Professor Barry Taylor, a Dunedin paediatrician and a member of the CDA board, suggested the possibility of analysing for the harmful elements a number of cot death post-mortem samples which he has available.

Riripeti Haretuku is one of the Maori cot death workers mentioned already. For some time she has been associated with efforts to lower the Maori cot death rate and in late 1995 she was elected to the board of CDA. It didn't take her long to size up the attitude of CDA towards the Richardson hypothesis. She suggested to the board that I be invited to discuss the issue with them but the reaction surprised her: a vehement refusal. To a newcomer who had no inkling of the staunch opposition to the hypothesis, it was astonishing. She telephoned me, wanting to find out more, and was patently interested in the research.

But CDA aren't the only players in the cot death arena. Other babycare professionals keep a close eye on cot death issues, and their attitudes to the hypothesis range from sincere interest to total acceptance.

Dr Pat Tuohy, policy director of the Royal New Zealand Plunket Society Inc, has been most cooperative, providing technical information and assisting with the testing of mattresses.

In February 1996 the Auckland branch of the New Zealand College of Midwives adopted mattress-wrapping as a matter of policy and recommended it to their national executive. This was followed in March by a request from the Antenatal Education Unit at North Shore Hospital for data on mattress-wrapping, and in May by an invitation to address the hospital midwives at National Women's Hospital.

In their March 1996 newsletter the Maternity Services Consumer Council published a lengthy article summarising the cot death debate, detailing the mattress-wrapping procedure, and concluding:

> It is important for families with young babies to be given sufficient information on the issue to enable them to decide whether they wish to follow or ignore Dr Sprott's advice regarding covering cot mattresses with polythene.

This is the very antithesis of CDA's policy. And not only the Maternity Services Consumer Council have seen the point about the right of parents to know. Since late 1995, *New Zealand Baby*

& *Child* and *North & South* have published feature articles on the hypothesis and *New Zealand Doctor* has given it prominent space. New Zealand Press Association journalist John Callan wrote a comprehensive article which was taken up by a large number of provincial newspapers. TV3 produced a short news documentary, again focusing on parents' right to know and to make up their own minds on mattress-wrapping.

The general public aren't convinced by CDA either. Since 1995 Red Nose Day, in-depth talkback radio programmes have highlighted the level of public disquiet, as have the hundreds of telephone calls which I have received.

There is a sense, however, in which CDA's stance doesn't actually matter any more. The impact of the groundswell of informed public opinion is that CDA are being marginalised. The focus of the cot death issue has moved, but CDA – just like FSID in Britain – remain stuck in a rut of their own making.

When it comes to solving the cause of cot death, CDA have become almost irrelevant.

15

The Mattress Suppliers

B arry Richardson's 1989 announcement of his findings put the British cot mattress industry on the spot. They were faced with an immediate public dilemma.

If, on the one hand, they took notice and modified their mattresses as Barry recommended, this would be interpreted by the public as an admission that previous mattresses had been faulty in some way. This could lead to an official requirement that mattresses be recalled; it would certainly lead to parents demanding free replacement mattresses or a cash refund; it might even result in legal claims for damages where babies had died – all unpalatable prospects for the manufacturers.

If, on the other hand, they ignored it and then the hypothesis was later officially recognised, the prospect was even less palatable: they could be faced with all the above, and also be accused of recklessly risking babies' lives by not taking appropriate action when they first learned of the matter.

But there was a third option: to take Richardson's advice, remove the offending elements, but say nothing about it. Which is precisely what several British manufacturers did. (One had commissioned a publicity campaign advertising their new 'chemical-free' mattresses, but lost their nerve at the last moment and didn't take the risk of running the advertisement with its possible implication that previously their mattresses had been unsafe.)

The easiest element to get rid of was antimony. Long regarded as one of the safest fire retardants, it had been incorporated for this purpose in PVC mattress materials since

1951 and by the 1980s was present in virtually all PVC used in cot mattresses. PVC cot mattress coverings had been introduced in Britain in 1948–49, and the amount of antimony in the PVC had been steadily increased over the years, most recently in response to the enhanced fire retardancy mandated by the Furniture and Furnishings (Fire Safety) Regulations 1988. The Department of Trade and Industry had given manufacturers four years' advance warning of the new Regulations and during this period all cot mattress manufacturers using PVC had moved towards the new standard.

It is noteworthy that the cot death rate in England and Wales increased from 1953 onwards, in parallel with the increasing concentration of antimony in PVC, and reached a peak in 1986–1988 of 2.3 deaths per 1000 live births.

In the late 1980s the Baby Products Association had strenuously lobbied the Government to have antimony removed from baby mattresses but had been overruled. In 1991 further concern was expressed, this time by the Turner Committee, who recommended that the need for additives (such as plasticisers and fire retardants) in cot mattresses should be carefully considered, and that if antimony trioxide was used as a fire retardant, only those grades containing the lowest possible levels of arsenic should be used. The Department of Trade and Industry, which is responsible for mattress safety, asked the British Standards Institution to adopt this latter recommendation into their cot mattress standard, BS1877 Part 10.

The Government had previously recognised the danger of a baby ingesting antimony but thought it had closed this loophole by means of BS1877 Part 10, which included a maximum level for soluble antimony in mattresses. They believed that the bulk of the antimony in a mattress, being insoluble, was not accessible to the baby. What they overlooked was the conversion of any antimonial compound by fungal activity to stibine, which the baby would then inhale. Furthermore, the Government did not regulate the incorporation of the even more dangerous phosphorus compounds in mattresses.

The Furniture and Furnishings (Fire Safety) Regulations 1988 were the culmination of the Government's concern over the effect of toxic gases released when household furniture was ignited. They are wide-ranging and increased the stringency of previous furniture safety Regulations. Mothercare lobbied the Government for the exclusion of nursery furniture from the 1988 Regulations and some relaxation was allowed, but the requirement for cot mattresses was retained.

Nevertheless, in response to Barry Richardson's publicity and despite the contrary opinion of the Government, Relyon and Mothercare suspended sales of mattresses containing antimony, and by the end of 1991 antimony had been removed from many cot mattresses in Britain. This, combined with the increased use of new mattresses and mattress-wrapping, was unquestionably responsible for most of the 73% reduction in the British cot death rate from 2.3 per 1000 live births in 1986–88 to about 0.62 in 1994.

Arsenic was quite rare in British mattresses, but interestingly it was the possibility of arsine generation which first drew Richardson's and Mitchell's attention to the potential hazard to babies posed by mattresses. In January 1989 Peter Mitchell had suggested to the Department of Health that arsenic could be implicated in cot deaths.

He and Richardson later discovered that where arsenic was present, normally this was only in trace amounts as an impurity in antimony which had been added to the mattress. Therefore, elimination of this antimony would get rid of the arsenic as well.

There was one exception to this: as already mentioned, Army-issue cot mattresses contained arsenic in the form of an arsenical biocide (OBPA), but having learned of the danger of arsine, the Army withdrew these mattresses and discontinued the use of OBPA.

The message about phosphorus did not get through as well, and in any event it was more widespread and more difficult to eliminate than antimony. Antimony was added for two purposes only, as a fire retardant in PVC and as a catalyst in polymer production, so removing antimony was no problem. Phosphorus, on the other hand, is present in several natural and synthetic materials used in cot mattresses, such as PVC, cotton and synthetic fabrics (including net) and certain plastic foams.

But overall the outcome was pleasing. Together, the purchase of new mattresses, covering of old ones, and removal of antimony from PVC led to the first recorded reduction in the British cot death rate. It fell by 38% in $2^{1/2}$ years. FSID would later try to take the credit and say that 'Back to Sleep' was the reason, but 'Back to Sleep' hadn't been heard of at that stage in Britain. Two years were to elapse before the British Department of Health belatedly adopted it.

At the time of writing, antimony in cot mattresses is almost a thing of the past in Britain. Manufacturers have been quietly eliminating phosphorus – although not publicising the fact – and most suppliers are believed to have eliminated it by December 1995.

The phosphorus remaining in many older mattresses is the reason why the cot death rate in Britain has levelled out. Admittedly the rate in Britain is low, but it is not dropping. 'Back to Sleep' augmented the success achieved by removing antimony, but 'Back to Sleep' doesn't work well against phosphine. Only when phosphorus is also eliminated will British cot mattresses be safe.

As previously noted, it is open to cot death parents in Britain to sue cot mattress manufacturers for damages under the Consumer Protection Act 1987.

The recently introduced General Product Safety Regulations 1994, implementing a European Community Product Safety Directive on general product safety, focus further attention on manufacturers' liability. Under these Regulations it is an offence for a producer to place on the market a product which is not safe.

The Regulations also require producers to carry out their own studies to determine whether their products are safe and, where necessary, to recall products from the market. Furthermore, the standard of acceptable risk is higher where products are for use by children.

British cot mattress manufacturers, therefore, do not have the luxury of waiting for the outcome of the Limerick Committee investigations if there is reason to suspect that their mattresses could be dangerous in normal use. Indeed the onus is on manufacturers to prove that there is no risk. Nor is it necessary to prove that a particular mattress has caused a cot death; simply the risk of cot death is sufficient to render the mattress unsafe under the Regulations.

The Regulations also impose on manufacturers a responsibility to monitor the safety of their products and to provide consumers with information so that they can assess the risk involved in using a product. For their part, retailers must pass this information on to buyers and also participate in the monitoring process.

In retrospect, the retention of cot mattresses within the ambit of the Furniture and Furnishings (Fire Safety) Regulations 1988 was a mistake, and not only because of Barry Richardson's findings about toxic gas generation from antimony and phosphorus. There was also an increase in the number of fatalities resulting from fires in bedding materials, probably because the more fire retardant there is in a burning mattress, the more toxic will be the fumes produced.

As the managing director of Tomy put it in late 1991: 'It's extraordinary that the Government should allow such potentially lethal chemicals into mattresses in such stark contrast to the Government directives on toys.'

In fact, the situation came about as the result of a series of errors and omissions. The use of PVC in cot mattresses brought organochlorine compounds into the baby's environment. When these compounds burn, very toxic gases result; so burning had to be controlled by the incorporation of a fire retardant. Antimony and phosphorus were the cheapest and most effective fire retardants, but their incorporation in mattresses introduced a source of virulent poisons. Also, PVC films require plasticisers to keep them flexible. The cheapest and most effective plasticisers contain phosphorus, source of an even more virulent poison. Furthermore, plasticisers are vulnerable to certain micro-organisms, especially in tropical climates, and the most effective biocide contained arsenic, source of the most virulent poison of the group.

The British Government unwittingly went along with all this, but regardless of the history, the ball is now firmly in the manu-facturers' court.

By the time the Richardson hypothesis made news in New Zealand after the first *Cook Report* programme, the whole emphasis was on antimony. So when Shirley Tonkin made her sweeping statement about New Zealand mattresses being free of antimony, not only was she wrong – she was also missing a vital point. Even if they were free of antimony (which some aren't), what about phosphorus and arsenic? Nevertheless the New Zealand mattress manufacturers heaved a collective sigh of relief. After all, here was the Cot Death Association itself reassuring them and the public that there was nothing to worry about.

Knowing as an industrial chemist that mattresses couldn't be pronounced absolutely safe without chemical analysis, I wasn't convinced. Specific information about mattress components was essential.

I asked everyone I could think of whether their particular products contained any phosphorus, arsenic or antimony: suppliers of mattress components both in New Zealand and overseas, companies importing components into New Zealand, flexible foam manufacturers, manufacturers of other mattress fillings, the cot mattress manufacturers themselves, the New Zealand Wool Board and the Wool Research Institute, and so on.

Keen to interest people in my research, I told them why I was asking: that these particular elements in mattresses had been conclusively linked to cot death.

For the most part, my enquiries were ignored. Some who responded didn't know what was in their product, and weren't interested in finding out anyway. Others denied that their products contained any of the elements, but couldn't back this up with analytical data. A few became quite hostile, but overall the mattress industry shrugged its shoulders.

This was no surprise: after all, Shirley Tonkin's views had been well publicised, and she had rubbished the hypothesis. Even if the industry's products did contain these substances, so what? The whole idea that the elements were causing cot death was crazy anyway.

There were, however, some bright spots. Lionel Bulcraig, an Auckland entrepreneur, is an inventor with an eye on the export market. In 1994 he was in the process of developing a new and imaginative concept in cots, and when he heard about Richardson's discovery, he wasn't prepared just to write it off. Realising the possible impact of the hypothesis on the safety of his new product, he promptly asked me for advice and equally quickly had his proposed cot mattress components analysed. It was just as well: much to his surprise (and that of the analyst he employed), both phosphorus and antimony were found in quantity. Thereupon he located materials which he could be certain didn't contain the elements, based upon the good quality assurance practices of the manufacturer.

For Lionel Bulcraig it was an important step in the development of his new product, one which he was sure would have both product safety and marketing benefits. For me there was an additional significance: it was proof positive that cot mattresses already on the market in New Zealand could (and probably did) contain one or more of the elements.

Another encouraging response came from an established New Zealand cot mattress manufacturer whom I contacted in late 1995. At first, it wasn't easy to gain their interest – the managing director told me quite openly that he had listened to Shirley Tonkin's assurances and believed them. Still, he heard me out and agreed that I had made a strong case which he couldn't ignore. In early 1996 he had all his cot mattress components analysed by the same analyst who had carried out the *Cook Report* testing in Britain.

But the question remained: why, despite CDA's publicity, did the New Zealand cot death rate remain static, the highest in the world?

The reason appeared evident – phosphorus primarily, with some contribution from arsenic and antimony arising mainly in natural products. Clearly, the New Zealand manufacturers couldn't provide a definitive answer regarding these elements, so mattresses had to be analysed – lots of them. Analysis would preferably encompass mattresses from different manufacturers, and would include mattresses in three categories: new, used, and (if I could obtain them) some on which babies had died of cot death.

Used mattresses were plentiful: there is a ready second-hand market. Cot death mattresses are more difficult to obtain, for a variety of reasons. New mattresses, of course, can be bought off the shelf but they can be quite expensive, and these ones were to be cut up for analysis! Here I met with a most rewarding and encouraging response. I visited the head office of The Baby Factory, a nationwide retailer of babycare items, and selected a wide range of typical cot mattresses and mattress overlays. This was a retail store, so I fully expected to pay for the items, but the managing director, having been told of the purpose, donated them on the spot!

A total of 66 cot mattress samples were sent to public analyst Ron Rooney in Basingstoke, to be analysed for phosphorus, arsenic and antimony.

The analytical results, which appear on pages 178–179, cover new products, used products and cot death baby bedding. They provide the answer to New Zealand's continuing and static cot death rate. To those who believe that the poisonous gas hypothesis has no relevance in New Zealand because the elements concerned are not present in New Zealand mattress materials: please study the analytical results.

New products

- Of 14 mattresses and mattress materials (2 imported) supplied by 12 manufacturers, only 1 item, a bassinet mattress, was free from the elements phosphorus, arsenic and antimony.

- Excluding the bassinet mattress, all the new products analysed contained phosphorus, 2 in excess of 500mg/kg. Six of the new items contained antimony, 2 in excess of 200mg/kg; and 2 items contained a small but measurable amount of arsenic.

- Two sheepskin rugs were analysed. These contained the highest concentrations of phosphorus and smaller amounts of both arsenic and antimony.

- Ti-tree bark contained a significant amount of phosphorus.

From these results it appears that virtually all the new cot mattresses and related products on sale in New Zealand are capable of generating one or more of the gases phosphine, arsine and stibine.

Used products

- The results showed a pattern similar to that for the new products, except that the concentrations of phosphorus were even higher.

- Sheepskin and coconut fibre contained the highest overall proportion of the harmful elements.

Cot death baby bedding

- The results were compiled from analysis of bedding components of 5 babies which had died of cot death. All 5 babies had been exposed to a high level of phosphorus, 4 to a relatively high level of antimony; and 3 to a measurable level of arsenic.

SCHEDULE OF ANALYTICAL RESULTS

Mfr	New products	phosphorus	arsenic	antimony
A	Waterproof wool mattress cover	+++	−	−
A	Bassinet mattress (polyester inner)	++	−	+++
A	Bassinet mattress (foam inner)	−	−	−
B	Imported PVC cot sheet	+++	−	−
C	PVC-lined cotton mattress protector	++	−	−
D	Acrylic underblanket	+	−	−
E	Sheepskin baby rug	+++++	+	++
F	Lambskin rug	+++++	+	+++
G	Ti-tree bark bassinet mattress	+++	−	−
H	Innersprung cot mattress	++	−	−
I	Ventilated cot mattress	++	−	++++
J	Kapok	++++	−	−
K	Innersprung cot mattress	++++	−	++++
L	Imported innersprung mattress	+++	−	+

No.	Used products			
1	Sheepskin baby rug	+++++	+	+++
2	Bassinet mattress	++++	−	−
3	Innersprung mattress	+++++	−	−
4	Foam mattress	++++	−	−
5	Foam mattress	+++++	−	−
6	Innersprung mattress	+++++	−	+
7	Coconut fibre	++++++	+	−
8	Foam mattress	++	−	−
9	Reconstituted foam mattress	+++++	−	−
10	Innersprung mattress	++++	−	+
11	Innersprung mattress	++++	−	+
12	Innersprung mattress	+++++	−	+++
13	Innersprung mattress	++++	−	−
14	Innersprung mattress	+++	−	−
15	Innersprung mattress	+++++	−	−

No.	Cot death baby bedding	phosphorus	arsenic	antimony
CD1	Pillow cover	++	−	−
CD1	Pillow polyester inner	+	−	+++
CD2	Mattress cover	+++	−	−
CD2	Mattress foam	++	++	−
CD3	Mattress cover	+++	−	−
CD3	Mattress foam	+++	+	−
CD3	Sheepskin rug	++++++	+	++++
CD4	Mattress cover	+++	−	−
CD4	Mattress foam	−	−	−
CD5	Mattress foam	+	−	−
CD5	Mattress cover	+++++	−	−
CD5	Sheepfleece underlay	+++	−	
CD5	Sheepskin rug	+++++	+	+++
CD5	Wool blanket	++	−	−

```
    −      =   not detected (<10mg/kg)
    +      =    10 ~ 50mg/kg
   ++      =    51 ~ 100mg/kg
  +++      =   101 ~ 200mg/kg
 ++++      =   201 ~ 500mg/kg
+++++      =   501 ~ 1000mg/kg
++++++     =   >1000mg/kg
```

While the analytical results for phosphorus and arsenic in the samples did not surprise me, I had not expected antimony to show up so frequently in New Zealand cot bedding, nor in such high quantity. Antimony was found in polyester products, in which it is often used as a catalyst, and also in all the sheepskins.

On the face of it, there would appear to be an anomaly in that the quantities of the elements found in some cot death bedding are lower than in some non-cot death items. This apparent anomaly was also encountered by Barry Richardson, who explained that concentrations of the elements in cot death bedding are often somewhat low compared with similar new products because during use of the mattress the elements have been dispersed as gases through biodeterioration.

The statement by CDA that the gaseous poisoning hypothesis does not apply in New Zealand because the harmful elements are not present in New Zealand cot mattress materials is patently wrong. There can be no doubt that the widespread incidence of compounds of these elements in the bedding of New Zealand babies is the cause of the exceedingly high cot death rate in this country.

From these analyses it appears that the same applies in Australia. At least two of the new products analysed were imported from Australia, and it was found that one of these contained a high proportion of antimony and both contained very high levels of phosphorus. Furthermore, the use of sheepskins and ti-tree bark mattresses is common in Australia.

One Australian manufacturer of mattress componentry whom I approached for information on this topic first tried to deny that their products contained any of the elements, but persistent questioning revealed that both phosphorus and antimony were present.

In 1994 the Executive Director of the Canadian Foundation for the Study of Infant Deaths told me that Canadian cot mattresses did not contain phosphorus, arsenic or antimony and claimed on this basis that the hypothesis had no application in Canada. However, this was contradicted by a major United States supplier to the Canadian cot mattress industry, who informed me that the use of phosphorus and antimony compounds was widespread over the whole of North America, Canada included.

Inquiries on this topic to retailers in Toronto met with a frosty reception, although one confirmed that they were aware that their mattresses contained antimony.

One of the arguments advanced *ad nauseam* against the gaseous poisoning hypothesis is that cot death has been known – albeit in smaller numbers – for many centuries, long before these chemicals were introduced into baby mattresses. But this argument is fallacious. The analytical results demonstrate that natural products which have been used historically for baby bedding, especially sheepskins, contain dangerous amounts of the elements. This same result would undoubtedly be obtained for the analysis of goatskins, which have also been used historically.

To reiterate: the schedule of results demonstrates that the problem element in New Zealand is phosphorus, just as it is in Britain now that antimony has been removed from most cot mattresses. Not only is phosphorus more difficult to eliminate from the cot environment; phosphine is the most dangerous of the three gases, being more toxic and less dense than stibine. Until the problem of phosphorus is recognised, the cot death rate in New Zealand will continue more or less as it is now.

The only immediate solution to the problem of cot death in New Zealand is to separate babies from the source of the poisonous gases, and this can be achieved only by the use of a non-toxic, gas-impermeable diaphragm such as a sheet of polythene or, if available, good quality surgical rubber. On no account should PVC be used for this purpose.

This advice applies equally to sheepskins. The use of these unprotected by polythene sheeting should be discontinued immediately.

16

Present and Future Policy

Ultimately, there can be only one policy regarding cot mattresses and the elements phosphorus, arsenic and antimony: to ensure that no mattress contains more than a minimal amount of any compounds of the elements. Such a change in manufacturing specifications would clearly take some time to achieve, but the following information will assist:

1 Materials containing nitrogen, phosphorus, arsenic or antimony should not be used. Biodeterioration of compounds of these elements (Group Vb) can generate the trihydrides ammonia, phosphine, arsine and stibine, and related compounds. Ammonia is lighter than air and disperses readily, but it is unpleasant, and degradation of nitrogen compounds such as melamine may severely damage mattress materials. Furthermore, nitrogen compounds tend to promote the growth of certain micro-organisms.

2 Neither phosphorus nor antimony fire retardants should be used.

3 Antimony trioxide should not be incorporated in organochlorine materials such as PVC.

4 If fire-retardant PVC is required, there are several effective non-toxic materials available, including aluminium oxide trihydrate (ATH), zinc borate, zinc stannate and zinc hydroxystannate. ATH is particularly suitable for fireproofing polyurethane foams.

5   Phosphorus-based plasticisers should be avoided. Phthalate plasticisers are common and do not cause cot death but certain questions have been raised about the safety of these additives. Further investigation of phthalate plasticisers is warranted. It may be preferable to use non-phthalate plasticisers such as epoxidised oils.

6   Biocides based on arsenic or phenyl phosphate should not be used. Instead, the addition of zinc soaps such as zinc octoate will protect against biodeterioration. Furthermore, a combination of zinc octoate and zinc borate will provide fire retardancy.

7   If green pigments are to be used, these must not be arsenical compounds (for example, Scheele's green or Paris green).

Proposed specification for cot mattresses and pillows

The following specification is proposed as a cot mattress standard:

i)   No amount of any compound containing any phosphorus, arsenic or antimony shall be added to any component of any mattress intended for use by infants.

ii) When tested by the standard analytical methods, there shall be no detectable phosphorus, arsenic or antimony.

iii) The lower limits of detection shall be stated in the analytical report and preferably should not be greater than:

   $0.001\% = 10mg/kg = 10$ parts per million.

iv) Any claim by a manufacturer that a cot mattress meets this requirement shall be supported by an analytical report to this effect from a recognised analytical laboratory.

v)   Any manufacturer of products to this specification shall maintain a quality assurance programme to ensure that the products continue to comply with the specification.

Cot mattresses complying with the above specification may display the **Campaign against Cot Death** logo.

Applications for permission to use the logo should be addressed to:

> T J Sprott
> 10 Combes Road
> Remuera
> Auckland 5
> NEW ZEALAND
>
> Phone: 64-9-523 1150
> Fax: 64-9-523 1150
> E-mail: sprott@iconz.co.nz

or to:

> B A Richardson
> Penarth Research International Ltd
> P O Box 142
> St Peter Port
> Guernsey
> CHANNEL ISLANDS GY1 3HT
>
> Phone: 44-1481-728559
> Fax: 44-1481-728559

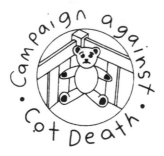

In Britain it has also been proposed that a new British Standard be established for cot mattresses and that complying mattresses should be of a specific colour and printed with a specific pattern to distinguish them from mattresses manufactured prior to the new Standard.

Each complying mattress should carry a label stating the manufacturer's name and address, the month and year of manufacture and batch number. The label should contain instructions for cleaning and state that 'This mattress is made from materials which do not contain more than 10mg/kg of phosphorus, arsenic or antimony.'

For manufacturers in New Zealand, it is probably almost impossible at present to produce cot mattresses which comply with the proposed specification for cot mattresses and pillows. The main difficulty will be to obtain cot materials which are free from phosphorus.

As to whether any of the elements are present in manufacturing materials, it is not sufficient to rely on information provided by suppliers unless:

1 The information is supported by a recent chemical analysis performed by an analyst who has demonstrated competence in determinations of this type on mattress materials; and

2 The supplier can provide proof of continuing adherence to the required specification, supported by some adequate quality assurance programme.

Mattresses not complying with the above specification

The immediate problem is the large number of existing mattresses currently or potentially in use, including stocks of unsold new mattresses and existing stocks of mattress componentry.

Of those cot bedding products currently on the New Zealand market which were included in the analytical programme, only one (a bassinet mattress) was found to comply with the proposed specification.

All mattresses which have not been shown to comply with that specification must be regarded as suspect.

Such mattresses should either be discarded or wrapped in a gas-impermeable diaphragm, the diaphragm known to be free from phosphorus, arsenic and antimony. Instructions for wrapping mattresses are printed inside the back cover of this book.

Proprietary mattress covers should not be used unless they comply with the above **Proposed specification for cot mattresses and pillows**.

Proprietary mattress covers complying with the specification may display the **Campaign against Cot Death** logo.

Proprietary chemical products

The New Zealand and Australian instructions for the use of these products should be modified to conform with the instructions for use of comparable products in Britain.

Nappy sterilants

The instructions should state that following soaking, the laundry is to be put through a full washing cycle.

Bottle and teat sterilants

The instructions should state that following soaking, bottles and teats are to be well rinsed in recently boiled and cooled water or in potable water.

17

Epilogue

On 23 August 1996 New Zealand will have another Red Nose Day. If last year is anything to go by, the sum donated will approach $1,000,000. Australia's Red Nose appeal will follow a week later, with anticipated donations of A$4,000,000. But after decades of research and hundreds of millions of dollars donated by the public in various countries, the cot death establishment still talk only about risk factors. And they don't even agree on those.

Take antimony, for example. In December 1994 Peter Fleming, Michael Cooke and Shireen Chantler (all members of the Limerick Committee) agreed with the Turner Committee that the use of antimony trioxide in cot mattresses should be seriously questioned. Ed Mitchell, on the other hand, stated in March 1995 that there was no evidence that antimony in cot mattresses was finishing up in babies.

Take bed-sharing. In July 1995 it was evident that Shirley Tonkin considered bed-sharing to be a risk factor *per se*. Not so the New Zealand Cot Death Association: according to them, this was her personal opinion; the Association hadn't decided whether to advise all mothers not to bed-share or only those who smoked (the same non-committal line taken by Peter Fleming in 1994).

Take smoking. In March 1995 Peter Fleming stated in effect that smoking by parents was the prime cause of cot death. To which Shirley Tonkin, when asked to comment, replied that she thought smoking probably exacerbated whatever *did* cause cot death – put another way, smoking was not the prime cause. But the New Zealand Public Health Commission had earlier stated that smoking *was* the prime cause of cot death.

Take mattresses coverings. In March 1995 Ed Mitchell said that mattresses should not be covered with polythene or rubber sheeting because babies might suffocate or become overheated. In the same month Peter Fleming said that babies were *safer* sleeping on plastic-covered mattresses. Then in June 1996 Lady Limerick followed Ed Mitchell's line that plastic-covered mattresses could lead to suffocation.

Take mattress-wrapping. In December 1994 the Foundation for the Study of Infant Deaths in Britain told parents, 'If you are worried [about cot death], wrap your mattresses.' But CDA and the Limerick Committee refuse to endorse mattress-wrapping.

What are parents to make of these discrepancies?

And the theories keep on coming. Take, for example, the latest from Canadian paediatrician Professor Dick van Velzen. Previously a researcher at the Children's Hospital Pathology Laboratory at Liverpool University and now back in Canada, he thinks he has found a virus which causes 50% of all cot deaths. He is busy developing a vaccine against this purported virus, which he estimates will take three years.

But how can the virus concept have any validity? Has he found a virus to which second babies are twice as susceptible as first babies, and third babies twice as susceptible as second babies, and to which first babies of wealthy parents are virtually immune?

In September 1995 Anne Diamond published a book, *A Gift From Sebastian – The Story of a Cot Death*. I scanned it with interest, expecting to find a ringing endorsement of the Richardson hypothesis. After all, only ten months previously she had informed millions of Britons that her baby had been poisoned. Instead, her 249-page book mentions the hypothesis in one brief paragraph just at the end.

She thanks Peter Fleming, Shirley Tonkin and Ed Mitchell 'and all the other brave, stubborn and talented people in [Britain] and elsewhere who cared enough to find out why our babies died – and, more importantly, what could be done about it.' But neither Peter Fleming nor Shirley Tonkin nor Ed Mitchell have found out why babies die of cot death, as they themselves admit. Barry Richardson has found out why, but he doesn't even rate a mention.

Nevertheless Anne Diamond goes on to inform the reader that she has covered her later baby's mattress with a protective cot sheet, 'just in case'. Perhaps she's not so convinced after all that the cot death establishment know what they're talking about.

And not just Anne Diamond. In May 1996 I was visited by Tim Burcher, Chairman of CDA. It was their first approach to me – an attempt to open a dialogue, as he put it. He was aware that a New Zealand manufacturer was having mattress components tested, and expressed the hope that the results would be provided to CDA. Why would CDA be interested, given their stated opinion of the Richardson hypothesis? Maybe they aren't quite so sure either.

June 1996 and the text of this book is complete, but the snippets of information continue to arrive.

From Barry Richardson comes fresh information about the sleeping position of cot death babies in Britain. In the days when antimony was a source of toxic gas, cot death babies were usually discovered lying face down. But now that antimony has gone, there is no apparent pattern of sleeping position when cot death babies are found: they can be face up or face down or lying on their sides. This stands to reason: the danger in Britain isn't stibine any more – it's phosphine, just as it is in New Zealand.

Meanwhile, the Limerick Committee continue their investigations, still chasing stibine. To focus on stibine is a pointless exercise now – mattress manufacturers in Britain removed antimony from their products long ago. The Committee should be focusing on phosphine.

On 10 June Lady Limerick had a meeting with three cot death mothers who are actively promoting the Richardson hypothesis. She told them that the Turner Committee hadn't demonstrated the generation of stibine – they referred her to the page in the Turner Report where its generation is documented. She told them that antimony was widespread in

THE COT DEATH COVER-UP?

households – they referred her to analytical reports to the contrary. She told one of the mothers, whose child had a high level of antimony in its hair (1200ng/g as compared with the mother's 47ng/g), that this was caused by the child lying on the sofa and other furniture – they burst out laughing.

The cot death establishment have arrived at their risk factors on the basis of epidemiology . But epidemiology only goes so far; at the end of the day, proposed solutions have to be tested in practice. For this reason both FSID and CDA set great store by 'intervention data', i.e. the practical result if you tell people to adopt a certain procedure. If the result is favourable, it is strong evidence that the idea was soundly based. This is what happened in New Zealand over face-up sleeping. When epidemiologists found that babies sleeping face down seemed to be at risk, they immediately told parents to put babies to sleep face up or on their sides, and then waited for the results. The 'intervention data' was not long in coming: face-up sleeping did reduce cot death. And it was this data which led to the introduction of 'Back to Sleep' in Britain.

To quote FSID Chairman Charles de Selincourt, intervention data is 'essential'. True. But FSID and CDA have excellent intervention data based on Richardson's recommendations: $2^{1}/_{2}$ years of falling cot death rate in Britain from June 1989 to December 1991, and beyond. Why don't they take note of this data and endorse mattress-wrapping? FSID and CDA may not be aware of it, but in June 1996 Lady Limerick admitted to Barry Richardson that her Committee hadn't been able so far to prove his hypothesis wrong.

And so back to New Zealand and the approaching Red Nose Day appeal. The publicity machine will swing into action, and once again New Zealanders will be treated to the sight of television personalities sporting red noses and to a jingle with a catchy tune. CDA will receive more largesse from the public – well-intended donations for cot death research.

But why should there be an appeal for further research funds? What is needed now is for CDA and others in the field of baby care to publicise mattress-wrapping; and for mattress manufacturers to eliminate phosphorus, arsenic and antimony from their products.

How long will this controversy go on? When will CDA and the cot death establishment act on the findings detailed in this book? We don't know. But as I said in the foreword, this book isn't written for the cot death establishment – it's written for the general public. They don't get research grants and they don't pore over medical journals, but they still get it right in the end.

To everyone involved in the care of babies – parents, grandparents, GPs, midwives . . . The cause of cot death has been established.

Wrap your baby's mattress.